HOW DO YOU KNOW IF IT'S RHEUMATOID ARTHRITIS?

- Do you suffer from morning stiffness (lasting at least 30 minutes)?
- Have you noticed swelling of the tissue around three or more joints?
- Do you have swelling of the tissue around joints in the hands or wrists?
- Do you suffer from symmetric swelling of the tissue around joints?
- Do you have nodules under the skin?
- Have you been told you have rheumatoid factor in the blood?
- Do X-rays reveal the erosion and/or loss of bone in the hand or wrist joints?

These are some of the indicators your doctor will use to make a diagnosis of rheumatoid arthritis—to learn what questions to ask and for the latest information read . . .

THE ARTHRITIS SOLUTION

THE
ARTHRITIS
SOLUTION

The Newest Treatments to Help You Live Pain-Free

ROBERT G. LAHITA, M.D., Ph.D.

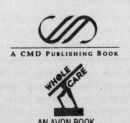

A CMD PUBLISHING BOOK

AN AVON BOOK

AVON BOOKS, INC.
1350 Avenue of the Americas
New York, New York 10019

Copyright © 1999 by CMD Publishing, a division of Current Medical Directions, Inc.
Illustration by Philip Ashley, C.M.I.
Published by arrangement with CMD Publishing, a division of Current Medical Directions, Inc.
Library of Congress Catalog Card Number: 99-94812
ISBN: 0-380-80778-5
www.avonbooks.com/wholecare

First WholeCare Printing: October 1999

WHOLECARE TRADEMARK REG. U.S. PAT. OFF. AND IN OTHER COUNTRIES, MARCA REGISTRADA, HECHO EN U.S.A.

Printed in the U.S.A.

WCD 10 9 8 7 6 5 4 3 2 1

~

Contents

~

Preface

There are periods in science and medicine when discovery is slow and progress is slow. This is the norm, and it is tolerated by both patients and doctors. However, there are also periods of prolific and rapid advance in not one, but many areas. This is the case at the end of the twentieth century for the family of drugs used to treat arthritic diseases. Chronic non-life threatening diseases do not have the social priority that diseases like breast cancer, AIDS, or heart disease have, yet these illnesses also take a great toll on human health and are as costly to our society.

The cause of the arthritic diseases and the very mechanisms that cause pain and inflammation to occur remain largely unknown. Despite this, the research and development of new medications is ongoing, and these new treatments are welcome and eagerly awaited. Those stricken with arthritis do not have the time or the luxury to wait long periods for these drugs. Doctors rejoice in telling patients what is to come and know that any delay in the availability of a new medicine results in long periods of patient suffering. Thus a book like *The Arthritis Solution: The Newest Treatments to Help You Live Pain-Free* serves an important role in providing the public with information about new and upcoming treatments.

In this book we address you—the patient—directly. In these pages, the new anti-inflammatory family of drugs called COX-2 inhibitors has garnered most of the attention. This is because they are new and useful and they demand both explanation and understanding. I am convinced that they will make a substantial difference to the care of persons with arthritis. We have not ignored the more traditional treatments and we put these in perspective throughout the book. Thus, the traditional non-steroidal anti-inflammatory drugs (NSAIDs) and the potent, and in some cases new, disease-modifying anti-rheumatic drugs (DMARDs) are also described. All treatments are explained in layman's terms in a question and answer format; these descriptions will help you understand what your doctor is talking about and will suggest questions that you may wish to ask.

Good communication between patient and doctor has always been an essential ingredient of health care, but short office visits may not always provide enough time for you to receive a detailed understanding of a new medication. Patient knowledge and openness between doctor and patient increases your awareness of your options and enhances the office visit, including that fragile and endangered entity called the "doctor-patient relationship." Maintaining this relationship is particularly important now as economic factors—such as cost controls and the growth of health maintenance organizations, or HMOs—have an increasing effect on your choice of doctors and treatments that will be covered by health plans.

Keeping patients out of the hospital is one of the doctor's goals today. It is likely that COX-2 inhibitors will have significantly reduced side effects compared to the traditional NSAIDs and thus lead to fewer hospital admissions. Rehabilitation, physical therapy, and psychological support will still be mandatory with any new agent, but money saved from reduced hospital costs can be put toward new research. Moreover, it is hoped that the huge savings from a decrease in the number of people on disability will be put toward research into the cause of these diseases and future drug development.

I thank many people for their contributions to this book. Most importantly I thank my able writer, Lisa Christenson, without whom this book would not have been possible. It is difficult to maintain research programs, see patients, teach, and write prolifically. Lisa has enabled me to appear to do the impossible. I also wish to thank Sarah Butterworth, Jennifer Mitchell, and Donna Balopole at CMD Publishing, where the development and initial editing of the book took place, and Ann McKay Thoroman of Avon Books for the initial idea for this book and her staff, who carried this book through to completion.

Robert G. Lahita M.D., Ph.D.
Saint Vincent's Medical Center
New York Medical College

ONE

What Is Rheumatoid Arthritis?

- Rheumatoid arthritis causes pain and swelling in the joints, typically the hands, feet, and hips.

- Rheumatoid arthritis can disfigure hands, paralyze joints, weaken the connective tissue in the heart and other vital organs, and create fatigue, depression, and severe pain.

- The symptoms of rheumatoid arthritis can flare up, causing pain for a period of time, and then disappear in 15% to 20% of patients. Sometimes, but rarely, they disappear for years.

- In most cases, rheumatoid arthritis gets worse over time, and should be treated early to prevent more damage to the affected joints.

- Several drugs are available that can relieve the pain and swelling associated with rheumatoid arthritis.

- Rheumatoid arthritis and related diseases afflict almost 37 million people in the United States, and that number keeps growing. The cost of treatment and lost productivity has been estimated to be as high as $50 billion per year in the United States alone.

• Between 43% and 85% of people with rheumatoid arthritis will be unable to work within 8 to 11 years after the disease begins. Almost 27% of patients are disabled within three years.

∾ CASE STUDY

Debra Jones, homemaker and mother, had just returned home from the hospital after the birth of her fourth child. "Congratulations! A girl at last!" exclaimed her friends and relatives. But Debra was so exhausted she could barely muster the enthusiasm expected of her. She knew it was not just the exhaustion of trying to perform all of her household chores while caring for her new baby and the rest of her family. She had lost a lot of blood during the delivery; maybe it was just that.

After four weeks of struggling to get through the days and nights with her new baby, Debra noticed that the joints in both of her hands and wrists were swollen and painful. As if that was not enough, the middle joint of each finger was swollen, making it difficult for her to use her hands. She was so weak that she could hardly lift the baby. Her toes were also swollen and her feet hurt so badly that she could hardly walk. When she went outside and it was chilly, not even really cold, she lost sensation in her fingers. She did not know what was happening—she had felt great during her pregnancy; why was this happening now?

Debra went to her family doctor, who performed a

complete physical examination. He found that the swelling and tenderness in her fingers and toes made her joints so painful that he could not even touch them. She complained that she felt stiff when she got out of bed—"It's like I've suddenly become an old woman"—and that this lasted for over an hour every morning. "How am I supposed to get three kids ready for school and change the baby's diaper when I can hardly move?" she asked. "My husband helps as much as he can, but he's trying to get ready for work!" It was not only the pain. Debra also had overwhelming exhaustion. "I feel like I'm dying of something," she claimed. "I pull my poor, stiff body out of bed and try to function, but it's like I'm moving through thick cotton instead of air."

Debra's doctor took X rays of her hands and wrists, which showed a lot of swelling of the tissue surrounding the joints. The bones of the joints had just started to erode, and the bones had begun to blanch (because of loss of bone tissue). Laboratory tests done on her blood showed a high level of rheumatoid factor and a high erythrocyte sedimentation rate.

Debra's diagnosis was early rheumatoid arthritis: morning stiffness, pain and swelling of the joints on both hands, and X-ray evidence of loss of bone tissue made this a fairly clear diagnosis. Her doctor prescribed an anti-inflammatory agent (ibuprofen) and a disease-modifying drug (methotrexate). He told her to be sure to rest until the drugs took effect and the pain went away.

The pain may subside, but the disease itself will not go away. Debra's doctor informed her that she would have to make a few changes in her life. He suggested that she get help caring for the children, especially the baby, as picking up the baby and doing the small manipulations necessary to feed and change a tiny baby put extra stress on joints. He recommended that a family member help out during the day, or that a babysitter be hired part time, if she and her husband could afford that; any household help would save wear and tear on Debra's joints. The doctor also suggested that Debra's husband take over the nighttime feedings so that Debra could be well rested, and that she nap when the baby napped, even if that meant leaving the laundry undone and the house messy. In general, the family would have to pitch in a little more with the household tasks that a stay-at-home mother usually does herself.

Debra's doctor also referred her to a physical therapist to set up an exercise plan to keep her joints moving and muscles strong without stressing the joints. He also suggested that she see an occupational therapist to help her figure out how best to perform the tasks at home, and how to allocate tasks to other family members so that she doesn't get too tired. He made an appointment for Debra to return in three months to check on the medication and her symptoms.

The presentation of Debra's disease is not an uncommon one. Rheumatoid arthritis often strikes women during the child-bearing years, and the symptoms are often masked during pregnancy. The disease can take a serious toll—it's not going to be easy for Debra to restructure her life, especially if her symptoms continue to get worse, with four small children and a household to take care of—but with the support offered by the physical and occupational therapists, and the continued vigilance of her doctor, Debra will be able to live a happy and productive life.

It was smart of Debra to go to the doctor while the disease was still in the early stages. Fortunately for her,

her doctor was knowledgeable about the diagnosis and treatment of rheumatoid arthritis and started her on methotrexate immediately. Starting on a disease-modifying drug such as methotrexate before a lot of damage has occurred can prevent irreversible changes in the joints and may mean that Debra will not become disabled.

What is rheumatoid arthritis?

Rheumatoid arthritis is a disease that causes inflammation, or pain and swelling, in the joints. Joints are the parts of your body where bones meet, such as the knee or hip. The ends of the bones are covered by smooth, tough cartilage, which keeps the ends of the bones from rubbing together. The entire joint, including the ends of the two bones, is enclosed within a capsule, which is lined with a special tissue called the synovium. The synovium produces synovial fluid, which fills the space between the two bone ends and helps the joint move smoothly. Muscles and tendons attach to the bones, supporting the joint and helping it to move. In arthritis, the synovium becomes inflamed, causing pain, stiffness, warmth, redness, and swelling.

Early in the disease, people may feel general fatigue and soreness, stiffness, and aching in the muscles—it may feel like having the flu. Unlike the flu, however, rheumatoid arthritis also causes pain in the joints, and the same joints on both sides of the body are usually affected. Pain or stiffness is usually first noticed in the hands or feet.

What causes rheumatoid arthritis?

It is not clear what causes this disease. Many people believe that rheumatoid arthritis is caused by changes in the weather, and that people living in cold, damp climates are more likely to get this disease. This theory, however, has been shown to be wrong—it does not make any difference where you live or what the weather is like. You are equally likely to develop rheumatoid arthritis whether you live in the hot, dry southwestern United States or cold, damp New England.

Researchers now believe that an infection like a virus or bacterium may trigger the start of rheumatoid arthritis in people who have a genetic tendency for the disease. There is an inherited component to the disease, although no clear genetic linkage has been identified. Most people with rheumatoid arthritis have a certain genetic marker, called HLA-DR4, but this marker is found in 10% to 15% of people in the United States, not all of whom develop rheumatoid arthritis. There is some evidence that people with HLA-DR4 may develop the disease at a younger age than people without HLA-DR4.

Rheumatoid arthritis is one of several diseases called autoimmune diseases, in which a person's immune system attacks cells in the person's own body. Other autoimmune diseases include multiple sclerosis, lupus, and some forms of diabetes. Usually, the immune system recognizes cells in the person's body as "self" and invaders as "foreign," but in autoimmune diseases, for some reason this distinction becomes blurred.

The current theory is that certain proteins, called antigens, interact with the marker HLA-DR4 on cells in people that have HLA-DR4. These antigens may come from a specific virus or bacterium that has not yet been identified. When the antigens combine with the HLA-DR4, they trigger the immune response to go into action. Instead of a normal immune response that would eliminate the virus or bacterium, however, this combination triggers an immune response that attacks the person's own cells.

Sometimes my arthritis feels better and sometimes worse. Is this common?

Yes. Rheumatoid arthritis has what doctors call a "variable course," which means that the symptoms can flare up and then disappear, sometimes for months at a time. In some patients (10% to 25% of all patients with rheumatoid arthritis), the symptoms disappear after the first flare-up and then never return.

The symptoms of rheumatoid arthritis can be aggravated by physical injury to the joint, infection, physical exhaustion, or even worry or stress. It is important, therefore, to protect your joints from further injury, eat well, maintain a good exercise program, and try to minimize stresses in your life (See Chapter 8, "Living with Rheumatoid Arthritis"). It may be useful to talk with a social worker or clinical psychologist if you find that there are stresses in your life that you need help with.

Can rheumatoid arthritis be treated?

The symptoms of rheumatoid arthritis can be treated to reduce the swelling, relieve the pain and stiffness, and help keep the joints working normally. The first drug your doctor will prescribe for you will probably be an anti-inflammatory, such as a nonsteroidal anti-inflammatory drug (NSAID—e.g., aspirin or ibuprofen), or the new class of drugs called COX-2 inhibitors (see Chapter 2, "What Are COX-2 Inhibitors?" and Chapter 3, "Other Available Treatments for Rheumatoid Arthritis"). While these drugs do not affect the course of the disease, they are an important part of drug therapy for rheumatoid arthritis, as they can help relieve the pain and swelling.

The disease process can be slowed with disease-modifying antirheumatic drugs (DMARDs), such as hydroxychloroquine, methotrexate, or azathioprine (see Chapter 3, "Other Available Treatments for Rheumatoid Arthritis"), but the disease cannot be cured. It is important to begin treatment with DMARDs early to prevent too much damage to the joints.

It is also important to get exercise, eat well, and rest. You might feel a great sense of fatigue, which will force you to take several short rests during the course of the day. You might also feel lethargic if you are depressed about having rheumatoid arthritis, as a side effect of the drugs you are taking, or because you are not getting enough restful sleep. Be sure to tell your doctor about your sleep patterns, so he can determine if taking low doses of an antidepressant medicine for a short time will help you get back into good sleep patterns. You should be able to stop taking the antidepressant once the disease is under control and you are getting a good amount of exercise. (See Chapter 8, "Living with Rheumatoid Arthritis.")

Be sure to tailor your exercise program to your own needs and abilities—if you were quite active before the disease, you will probably be able to undertake more physical activities than if you were less active. In either case, however, it is important to get some exercise, and to balance exercise with rest. Tell your doctor if the pain is preventing you from getting enough exercise. It may be useful to see a physical therapist to design an exercise program, and to learn some exercises that can help with range of motion in the joints.

Will my disease get better or worse over time?

Rheumatoid arthritis is a degenerative disease, meaning that the symptoms worsen over time as the joint becomes progressively more damaged. The inflamed membrane can invade and damage nearby bone and cartilage, and the joint may lose its shape and alignment, resulting in pain, loss of movement, and, in some cases, destruction of the joint. About one person in six develops some crippling deformities as a result of rheumatoid arthritis.

As time goes by, the disease generally becomes less aggressive—you will feel less tired and stiff, and no new joints will be affected. The disease will not get any better, however, and you will have to live with the amount of pain and stiffness that you have.

How common is it?

Rheumatoid arthritis is very common. It affects 1% of the population of the United States, or 1 in 100 people. It affects about four times as many women as men, and symptoms are usually first noticed by people between the ages of 25 and 50. The symptoms often become much less severe if a woman becomes pregnant, but then they return after the baby is born. (See Chapter 8, "Living with Rheumatoid Arthritis," for more information on childbirth and rheumatoid arthritis.)

This disease seems to run in families, although it is not directly hereditary and there is no gene that causes rheumatoid arthritis. It does mean, however, that if your parents or grandparents have rheumatoid arthritis, you have an increased chance, but not an absolute certainty, of developing the disease. Likewise, if you have rheumatoid arthritis, your children are at increased risk, but unlike in the case of some inherited diseases, they will not necessarily develop the disease. There is no way of testing to see if you or your family members will get this disease.

Rheumatoid arthritis shows little preference for race or nationality—it occurs in all ethnic groups in all parts of the world.

Many famous people during the course of history and living today have had arthritis. The painter Peter Paul Reubens, who lived from 1577 to 1640, portrayed what was probably the progression of his own disease in the portraits he painted of his patrons. Other famous historical figures who suffered from arthritis include Christopher Columbus; Mary, Queen of Scots; Julius Caesar; and Pope Pius II.

Famous people living in our lifetime who have led successful and productive lives despite living with arthritis include former First Lady Betty Ford; actors Elizabeth Taylor, Katharine Hepburn, and James Garner; the dancer Martha Graham; football players Joe Namath and Dick Butkus; the surgeon Christiaan Barnard; and former President Ronald Reagan.

It may seem difficult and even overwhelming at the beginning, but like these famous people, you can learn to live with rheumatoid arthritis. The therapies available today, both medicines and physical therapy, can help you to cope with the symptoms of this disease and can make living with arthritis much easier.

I think I've heard of other kinds of arthritis. If that's true, what are the other types and what's the difference?

There are over 100 different kinds of arthritis and related conditions. A few of the most common are listed in Table 1.

Table 1. Diseases That Have Arthritis as a Major Manifestation

Rheumatoid arthritis
Osteoarthritis
Lupus erythematosus
Scleroderma (progressive systemic sclerosis)
Ankylosing spondylitis
Gout and pseudogout
Polymyositis
Polymyalgia rheumatica
Fibromyalgia (fibrositis)
Lyme disease
Gonococcal arthritis
Nongonoccal infectious arthritis
Rheumatic fever
Reiter's syndrome/reactive arthritis
Viral arthritis
AIDS arthritis
Juvenile rheumatoid arthritis
Tendonitis
Bursitis

ᖰ CASE STUDY

Jim O'Reilly is a 51-year-old banker. Never one to complain, he ignored the off-and-on pain in his knee for months as it got progressively worse. When he got home from work he watched the news, and then found himself limping for about a half hour after he got up. The knee pain had also begun to affect his favorite weekend activity, hiking with his wife, son, and daughter-in-law. On a recent weekend, he noticed that the pain was slight when they climbed up a small mountain, but was quite severe when they went down again. The next morning he could hardly straighten his leg.

Jim decided it was time to see a doctor. The doctor found some mild swelling around the knee, but little pain when she touched it, and it was not red and hot. The doctor anesthetized the knee with a local anesthetic, inserted a needle, and drew out some fluid. Jim was amazed at how painless the procedure was—when the doctor told him she was going to stick a needle in his knee, he imagined a sharp, shooting pain! The fluid was deep yellow colored, slightly cloudy, and thick. It was not so thick and cloudy that you could not read newsprint through it, and the doctor explained that this is important—if it was too cloudy, that could mean too many cells, which might indicate an infection. She also told him that there were about 1,000 white blood cells in 1 milliliter of fluid—that meant no infection. She also did not see crystals in the fluid, which there would be if his condition was gout.

Jim's knees were X-rayed. The X rays showed that the joint space was narrower than normal, with some thickening of the bone and some extra outgrowth of bone.

It was osteoarthritis, the most common type of arthritis. Jim's doctor prescribed acetaminophen and told him to take it easy on his knees. She also told him to call her office if the acetaminophen did not work and then she would start him on ibuprofen. She referred him to a physical therapist to help design an exercise program that would keep him flexible and fit without stressing his knees. She also suggested that he lose a few pounds— even though he was only about 10 pounds overweight, that 10 pounds could be hard on the knees. If his knee started to hurt, she recommended using a heating pad. She reassured him that if he took care of himself, his knee should not get any worse and he would be able to continue with his daily routine. No more strenuous hikes were permitted, however; in fact, no exercise was allowed that involved pounding of the knees. The doctor told Jim to return in one year, to check on the knee and to make sure no other joints had become involved.

I've heard of osteoarthritis. Is that similar to rheumatoid arthritis?

Osteoarthritis, also called degenerative arthritis or degenerative joint disease, is the most common type of arthritis. Osteoarthritis occurs when the cartilage that covers the ends of bones breaks down, leaving the bones exposed and causing pain and stiffness. Researchers are not sure what causes the destruction of the cartilage, but it seems to be related to changes in collagen and proteoglycans, two of the main components of cartilage. For some reason, the collagen network is changed and the cartilage in osteoarthritis contains much more water than normal cartilage. There is much less inflammation with osteoarthritis than there is with rheumatoid arthritis.

This disease usually affects the fingers and the weight-bearing joints, such as the knees, feet, hips, and back, and may be caused by stress or injury to the joint. Osteoarthritis affects many people as they get older, both men and women, and is most noticeable after the age of 45. Men tend to get this disease in their hips, women in their hands. Anti-inflammatory drugs, such as ibuprofen, can help alleviate the pain and swelling of osteoarthritis. Treatment of the affected joints with heat or cold, such as a heating pad or an ice pack, can also help. It is also important to continue to exercise, but not to stress the affected joints. Surgery may be necessary to alleviate the pain, or even to replace the joint if the osteoarthritis is advanced.

Are there drugs to stop the damage to the joints in osteoarthritis?

There is currently no treatment that will stop the destruction of cartilage in osteoarthritis. Researchers are working hard to find one, however, and some show promise. Some experiments have used preparations of the structural components of collagen. Another approach is to restore normal joint lubrication by injecting hyaluron, one of the components of synovial fluid. Other researchers are trying to prevent the enzymes that break down collagen from working.

I have a friend with lupus, and her symptoms are similar to mine. How do I know I don't have lupus?

Lupus erythematosus is a disease in which a person's immune system mistakenly attacks the body's own cells and tissues (autoimmune disease), causing inflammation that can be life-threatening. Lupus can affect the joints, skin, lungs, heart, kidneys, nervous system, and blood. Although the initial symptoms of lupus and rheumatoid arthritis may be similar, the two diseases can be readily distinguished by tests performed by your doctor.

This disease occurs in women ten times more often than men, and in African Americans more frequently than in whites. Symptoms often first appear between the ages of 18 and 45, and include a butterfly-shaped rash over the cheeks and across the bridge of the nose; scaly, disc-shaped sores on the face, neck, and/or chest; abnormal sun sensitivity; and arthritis. Treatments include the careful use of anti-inflammatory drugs, such as ibu-profen, and immunosuppressive drugs to slow down the hyperactive immune system. Examples of these drugs are cortisone, azathioprine, and cyclophosphamide. It is also important to eat well and balance rest with exercise—people with lupus tend to tire easily and must not overdo exercising.

Isn't there a form of arthritis that affects mostly the spine?

Ankylosing spondylitis is a form of arthritis that can affect the hips and shoulders as well as the spine. This disease occurs four times more often in men than in women. In women, ankylosing spondylitis is often mis-diagnosed as rheumatoid arthritis, which can lead to dis-astrous results. If not treated, ankylosing spondylitis can cause the spine and ribs to become rigid, making it dif-ficult to move and even to breathe. This disease is best treated with anti-inflammatory drugs and physical therapy.

My cousin has symptoms that sound like those of arthritis, but her doctor says it's something called fibromyalgia. What is fibromyalgia?

Fibromyalgia is a disease that affects the muscles and their attachments to bone. Fibromyalgia was first de-scribed more than 150 years ago, but as recently as the 1980s was often not taken seriously. Many doctors told patients that there was nothing wrong with them, or that their symptoms were psychological. Some people still believe that their symptoms are a normal sign of aging.

But the often overwhelming fatigue and widespread muscle pain that characterize fibromyalgia are not normal signs of aging. The muscle pain often shows up as tender trigger points, or certain areas of the muscle that are more sensitive to pain. Patients may also experience stiffness, especially in the morning, and may find it difficult to sleep restfully.

Fibromyalgia occurs in ten times more women than men, most often after the age of 40. The condition can be treated with low doses of antidepressant drugs and mild pain medicine, and the symptoms may improve with exercise and more sleep.

Isn't there an arthritis-like disease that is spread by ticks?

Lyme disease, which causes flulike symptoms and joint pain, is transmitted by ticks carrying the bacterium *Borrelia burgdorferi.* This disease occurs most often in southern New England and the mid-Atlantic states, the Midwest, and the West Coast of the United States. The best way to prevent Lyme disease is to wear protective clothing, to use insect repellant when walking in wooded or grassy areas, and to check yourself and your pets carefully after a walk to remove any ticks. The tick must be embedded under the skin in order to spread the disease, so if you can find them within a couple of hours, before they have embedded, you're safe.

The course of the disease varies greatly, but is generally characterized by flulike symptoms shortly after the tick bite. In most, but not all, cases, a characteristic "bull's eye" rash will surround the region of the bite, making it easy to know you have been bitten and should get treatment. Lyme disease can be readily treated with antibiotics to kill the bacteria, and anti-inflammatory drugs are given for the joint pain and swelling. If untreated, serious complications can occur that affect the joints, nervous system, and heart. A vaccine to prevent Lyme disease—LYMErix, manufactured by SmithKline Beecham—was approved by the FDA in December 1998, for use in people aged 15 to 70 years. Three doses of the vaccine, given over a year, provide a 78% protection rate against the disease. A second vaccine—ImuLyme, manufactured by Pasteur Mérieux Connaught—is awaiting FDA approval.

Is gout related to arthritis?

Most people don't think of gout as being related to arthritis, but it is. Gout is a painful joint disease that results when crystals form in the joints, often the big toes, ankles, and knees, causing pain and swelling. These crystals are made up of a natural substance called uric acid, which doesn't hurt the body in small amounts. In some people, however, the body either produces too much uric acid or produces the right amount but cannot get rid of it. After years of accumulating in the body, the excess uric acid collects in the joints and forms crystals, causing pain and inflammation.

This disease affects more men than women, and usually strikes after the age of 40. It may come on quite suddenly, after a long walk, a rich meal, or surgery. Treatments for gout include anti-inflammatory drugs, colchicine, and corticosteroids. Losing weight if you are overweight and not drinking too much alcohol can also help alleviate the symptoms. Although not caused by eating the wrong foods, the symptoms of gout can be aggravated by some foods, such as asparagus, gravy, herring, liver, mushrooms, mussels, and sardines, and these foods should be avoided.

Is osteoporosis related to arthritis?

Osteoporosis is not really related either to osteoarthritis or to rheumatoid arthritis—it's not an arthritis-like disease—but it is often found in patients with arthritis, for a variety of reasons. Osteoporosis is a bone disease in which the bones become brittle and break more easily because they have lost calcium. Osteoporosis is more severe in postmenopausal women, and is the cause of broken hips in one of every five women under the age of 75.

Osteoporosis can be prevented. Eating a diet with plenty of calcium and getting regular exercise are two easy steps you can take, and should take, even if you are young. A normal, healthy man should get at least 800 mg of calcium a day. Young women, women who are pregnant or nursing, postmenopausal women, and men over the age of 65 should get at least 1,500 mg per day. Most people do not get enough calcium every day, but it's easy to do, with a few small changes in your diet.

Try drinking three glasses of nonfat milk every day—that's only one glass with every meal. Cheese is good too, but it is higher in fat than milk. Yogurt is also an excellent source of calcium, and a good mid-afternoon snack. Other calcium-rich foods include almonds, broccoli, beans, kale, tofu, canned salmon, and canned sardines.

If you cannot change your diet to get enough calcium, you can take a calcium supplement, but it's not as good as getting calcium from foods.

Weight-bearing exercise, such as walking, is important in maintaining strong bones. Try to walk one half to one mile every day, or at least four miles a week. As good an exercise as swimming is, it is not weight-bearing, so don't include that in your four miles!

What are the first symptoms of rheumatoid arthritis?

Rheumatoid arthritis usually starts gradually. You might feel tired and achy, like you have the flu. Most people feel pain and stiffness in one or more joints, usually the hands, wrists, or feet. The joints may not be swollen at the beginning but will probably start to swell within a couple of months. The joint pain almost always occurs in symmetrical joints, that is, the same joints on both sides of the body. For example, you might feel pain in both wrists or in the same finger on both hands.

The above is the usual course of rheumatoid arthritis, but sometimes it varies. Some people do not get joint pain right away; they just feel stiff all over, especially when they get up in the morning. The stiffness usually lasts more than 30 minutes. Others feel achy and stiff, particularly in the hips and shoulders, and this may continue for weeks or months before the joints start to swell. This course of the disease occurs most often in older people and may be confused with a disease called polymyalgia rheumatica. Other people have swollen joints that are not painful at first. There is much variation in the symptoms of rheumatoid arthritis; however, a symmetric painful series of joints particularly in the hands, feet, and wrists is the most common presentation for this disease.

In some people, the joints are painful and swollen, then get better, then worse again. Rheumatoid arthritis can also, but very rarely, be asymmetric, that is, it can occur in a joint on one side of the body but not in the corresponding joint on the other side. Eventually, even in these people, the joints on the other side are also affected—the disease becomes symmetric, the typical course for rheumatoid arthritis.

Some people have severe disease right away—the disease starts off with several swollen, painful joints, and the person feels very tired and feverish and has no appetite.

Are there different classifications of rheumatoid arthritis, depending on how it starts and progresses?

Yes, rheumatoid arthritis has been classified into four different types: spontaneously remitting disease, remitting, remitting progressive, and progressive.

Spontaneous remission means that without treatment, or just with NSAIDs, the symptoms of the disease disappear. They may return later, and you may need to start taking NSAIDs again, but for a while you have complete relief. In rare cases, about 5% to 10% of people with rheumatoid arthritis, the symptoms never return.

Remitting disease means that the person has a series of flare-ups with a return to normal in between. This can be difficult to deal with, because it is not known when a remission is going to occur and when the symptoms will return. DMARDs (see Chapter 3, ''Other Available Treatments for Rheumatoid Arthritis'') may be needed to prevent permanent joint damage during the flare-ups.

People suffering from remitting progressive disease experience flare-ups but never quite return to feeling normal in between. There is a good chance that the joints will be damaged with this type of disease if DMARDs are not taken.

The person with progressive disease never experiences remissions or flare-ups, just a gradual increase in the pain, swelling, and joint damage over time. Usually the progression is slow, but in some cases one can become disabled quite quickly. It is very important to start taking DMARDs as soon as it becomes obvious that this is the course the disease is following.

Is there any way to tell how bad my disease is going to get?

It is not easy to predict how the disease will progress in any one person, but there are some factors that do correlate with a more or less favorable outcome. These are listed in Table 2. Some factors that were previously thought to be associated with more severe disease, such as having the marker HLA-DR4 in the blood, may not actually be related to more severe disease.

Table 2. Factors That Correlate with Prognosis

More Favorable Prognosis	Less Favorable Prognosis
Onset at a younger age	Rapid onset of symptoms
Absence of rheumatoid nodules	Onset at an older age
Absence of, or few, manifestations outside of the joints	High levels of rheumatoid factor early in the disease
Absence of rheumatoid factor	Early involvement of large joints
Male gender	Female gender
	Presence of rheumatoid nodules
	Early appearance of erosions in the joints
	Vasculitis
	Scleritis
	Manifestations outside of the joints

How serious is rheumatoid arthritis?

Rheumatoid arthritis can be very serious. Over time the joints become more and more affected, and the pain and limited movement can make the activities of daily living nearly impossible. If rheumatoid arthritis is not treated early, the joints can become permanently damaged and deformed.

That is why it is so important to see your doctor and begin treatment early (see Chapter 3, "Other Available Treatments for Rheumatoid Arthritis"). Early treatment with DMARDs, such as hydroxychloroquine or methotrexate, can slow or even halt the progression of the disease, preventing some of the joint damage that might occur. Treatment with anti-inflammatory drugs such as ibuprofen, naproxen, or other NSAIDs can alleviate the pain and swelling, allowing you to be more active. And physical therapy can help you develop an exercise program that is suitable for your abilities. It's important to keep exercising, to keep the joints moving and the muscles active.

The disease can also have profound psychological effects: Daily pain can cause increased stress and fatigue, which can lead to anger and depression. Medicines to alleviate the pain, combined with a reasonable exercise program, can help stave off stress and depression.

Does arthritis affect other parts of the body besides the joints?

Yes, and the complications that occur in other parts of the body, not the joints, are the most serious. These are called extra-articular manifestations of arthritis. Some of these complications, such as rheumatoid lung and inflammation of the blood vessels, can be fatal. Most of these are not common, however; fewer than 5% of people with rheumatoid arthritis develop the most serious complications of the disease. These complications can usually be minimized, or even prevented, by treating the disease promptly.

- About 15% of people with rheumatoid arthritis develop inflammation of the tear ducts and salivary glands, which causes them to have dry eyes and mouth. Your eyes may feel itchy or gritty. Use of eye lubricants, called artificial tears, can help. If your mouth is dry, be sure to brush your teeth, floss, and use an antiseptic mouthwash regularly. Lack of saliva can increase tooth decay.

- In very rare cases, inflammation of the tissues in the eyes, called ophthalmitis, can occur. This can lead to erosion of the eyeball, and, in the worst cases, the eyeball can become punctured, causing blindness. Be sure to tell your doctor if you have pain or redness in your eyes, or problems seeing.

- Involvement of the joints in the face, such as the jawbone, can make it difficult to open your mouth and cause severe pain in the temples. This problem should resolve with medication that treats the arthritis.

- Breathing discomfort develops in about 30% of people with rheumatoid arthritis, caused by arthritis in the joints between the collar bones and chest bone. This pain will also resolve with treatment.

- Rheumatoid lung is a condition whereby immune cells accumulate in the lung, causing inflammation of the lung. This can lead to troubled breathing, shortness of breath, and, in rare cases, death. Lung disease is not very common—a mild case occurs in 10% to 20% of people with rheumatoid arthritis—but it occurs more often in people who smoke cigarettes.

- Felty's syndrome is a very rare complication of rheumatoid arthritis—it occurs in less than 1% of people with longstanding disease. This syndrome is associated with a low number of white blood cells and an enlarged spleen, which means your body cannot fight off infections as well as it used to. Your platelet count might also be decreased, which means your blood will not clot as well and you run the risk of excessive bleeding. Skin ulcers and dark patches on the skin are other signs of Felty's syndrome. Felty's syndrome usually clears up after treatment with DMARDs. If it does not, you might have to have your spleen removed.

- Rheumatoid vasculitis, or inflammation of the blood vessels, usually occurs in people who have a high level of rheumatoid factor in their blood. Vasculitis can affect blood vessels in any part of the body. In mild cases, it prevents adequate blood flow to the skin, causing skin ulcers. These sores can be treated by washing carefully and gently with an antiseptic soap, and will clear up with DMARD treatment. If vasculitis affects the vessels in the brain, however, it is more serious—it can cause strokelike symptoms, and can be fatal. Vasculitis can also affect the arteries of the lung, heart, intestines, and kidneys, interfering with the normal functioning of these organs. Rheumatoid vasculitis can cause the small blood vessels in your hands, fingers, feet, or toes to become completely blocked up, preventing blood flow. The affected area may have to be amputated. The serious forms of rheumatoid vasculitis can be treated with corticosteroids or much stronger chemotherapeutic agents, or both in combination. These stronger agents are disease-modifying drugs (DMARDs) by definition.

- Rheumatoid nodules can appear as bumps in the skin, often on the hands, feet, or elbows. These nodules are unsightly but not dangerous. Nodules can also form on organs, such as the heart or brain, where they can interfere with normal functioning, but are rarely fatal. Nodules usually form in patients who test positive for rheumatoid factor in their blood. Nodules do not require any special treatment unless they are painful or become infected. If you have nodules, however, you should talk to your doctor about DMARD treatment, since their presence can indicate that your disease is getting worse.

- Mild anemia is found in one half to two thirds of patients with rheumatoid arthritis. Anemia can be the result of the long-standing inflammation in arthritis and indicates how severe the disease is. This type of anemia usually clears up with DMARD treatment. Anemia can also develop as a side effect of NSAID treatment, because NSAIDs irritate the stomach lining and cause bleeding. If you have this type of anemia, you might have to stop taking NSAIDs in order to get your red blood count back up to normal.

In some cases, side effects of the drug therapies used to treat rheumatoid arthritis can be similar to complications of the disease itself. For example, treatment with methotrexate can produce rheumatoid nodules that are treatable. Your doctor will conduct tests to tell the difference.

What joints does rheumatoid arthritis affect?

Rheumatoid arthritis usually first affects the joints in the wrists, hands, knuckles, feet, and toes. As the disease progresses, it may also affect the shoulders, elbows, hips, and knees. (See illustration.) The spine is affected in about 40% of all people with rheumatoid arthritis, usually in the section between the shoulder blades and the base of the skull. You might feel severe, blinding pain when you move your neck, or pain and tingling down your arms when you tilt your head backward.

The joints most often affected in the hands are the middle knuckle of the finger (proximal interphalangeal, or PIP, joint), the knuckle where the finger meets the hand (metacarpophalangeal, or MCP, joint), and the wrist (carpometacarpal, or CM, joint). The two knuckles of the thumb—the MCP joint and the interphalangeal (IP) joint—can also be affected. In the foot, the knuckles of the toes—the PIP joint (closest to the ankle) and the distal interphalangeal, or DIP, joint (farthest from the ankle)—are often affected, as is the metatarsophalangeal (MTP) joint, where the big toe connects to the foot.

The main thing doctors look for in diagnosing rheumatoid arthritis is pain in the same joints on both sides of the body, for example, both wrists or the same knuckles on both hands. Another signpost of rheumatoid arthritis is stiffness in the joints first thing in the morning and lasting 30 to 60 minutes or longer. Other diseases can cause one or the other of these symptoms, but if you have both, chances are it is rheumatoid arthritis. For example, fibromyalgia causes morning stiffness, but the pain is more muscular and may not be symmetrical. Osteoarthritis affects some of the same joints as does rheumatoid arthritis, but the pain may not be symmetrical.

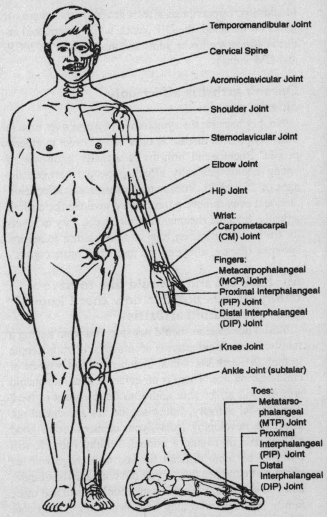

Temporomandibular Joint

Cervical Spine

Acromioclavicular Joint

Shoulder Joint

Sternoclavicular Joint

Elbow Joint

Hip Joint

Wrist:
Carpometacarpal
(CM) Joint

Fingers:
Metacarpophalangeal
(MCP) Joint
Proximal Interphalangeal
(PIP) Joint
Distal Interphalangeal
(DIP) Joint

Knee Joint

Ankle Joint (subtalar)

Toes:
Metatarso-
phalangeal
(MTP) Joint
Proximal
Interphalangeal
(PIP) Joint
Distal
Interphalangeal
(DIP) Joint

Location and names of joints. In rheumatoid arthritis, the joints in the
wrists, fingers, and toes are usually affected first (see text).

In addition, osteoarthritis affects generally the outermost joints on the hand, the DIP joints, while rheumatoid arthritis affects the lower joints and the wrists (PIP, MCP, and CM joints).

Doesn't arthritis afflict only elderly people?

No, but because the symptoms get worse over time in most people, the disease is often most severe in elderly people. Rheumatoid arthritis is actually a disease of young adults, generally affecting people between the ages of 25 and 50. Rheumatoid arthritis can affect children and even infants, a form called juvenile rheumatoid arthritis. Juvenile rheumatoid arthritis can vary in severity from mild, affecting four or fewer joints, to severe, systemic disease, affecting the joints and other organs.

My husband and I would like to have a family. Is this possible now that I know I have rheumatoid arthritis?

Yes! Your disease should not stop you from having a family. Rheumatoid arthritis occurs most often in people in their 20s and 30s, which includes a lot of women of child-bearing age. There is no evidence that rheumatoid arthritis will affect your ability to get pregnant or have a successful delivery. Likewise, the disease should not affect the developing fetus—your chances are as good as anyone's of having a normal, healthy baby. It will probably be more difficult for you to manage with an infant and a toddler than if you did not have the disease, and you should discuss this with your husband and other family members who may be called upon to help care for your young children (see Chapter 8, "Living with Rheumatoid Arthritis").

Your disease might even get better during pregnancy, which is good, since you might have to stop taking DMARDs while you're pregnant—some DMARDs cause birth defects (see Chapter 3, "Other Available Treatments for Rheumatoid Arthritis"). Be sure to tell your doctor of your plans before you stop using birth control so you can decide what is the best course of action for you to take.

Should I go to the doctor if I suspect that I have rheumatoid arthritis, or should I wait until the pain is pretty bad?

It is important to see a doctor early if you think you might have rheumatoid arthritis. Early treatment with DMARDs may prevent the symptoms from progressing as rapidly (see Chapter 3, "Other Available Treatments for Rheumatoid Arthritis"). DMARDs are drugs such as hydroxychloroquine, methotrexate, and azathioprine that slow, and may even halt, the progression of the disease. Until recently, most doctors held off treating patients with DMARDs until the disease was fairly far along. Now, however, doctors have begun to treat patients very early with DMARDs, to prevent irreversible damage to the joints. It is important, therefore, to obtain a diagnosis as soon as possible, so you can begin treatment.

Your doctor can also get you started on the best medication available to treat the pain and swelling. These medicines include NSAIDs (see Chapter 3, "Other Available Treatments for Rheumatoid Arthritis") and, now, the COX-2 inhibitors, a new form of NSAID (see Chapter 2, "What Are COX-2 Inhibitors?"). You can get many NSAIDs at a pharmacy without a prescription, but it is a good idea to consult a doctor first, since you might be taking medicine for a long time (even the rest of your life), and you want to make sure you have the most appropriate one.

See your doctor if you have:

- Pain and stiffness in the morning

- Pain, tenderness, or swelling in one or more joints

- Recurrence of pain, especially in more than one joint

- Recurrence of pain in the neck, lower back, knees, and other joints

Rheumatoid arthritis should be treated early to prevent irreversible damage to the joints. See your doctor if you have these symptoms so you can start treatment.

Are there tests to determine if I have rheumatoid arthritis?

Yes, there are tests that can determine if you have the disease. The most important factor in diagnosing rheumatoid arthritis is a good medical history and physical examination. Your doctor should examine all parts of your body, including your eyes, lungs, heart, and throat. Rheumatoid arthritis and related diseases affect the entire body, not just the joints, and it is important for your doctor to get a good idea of the whole picture.

Feeling stiffness in the joints in the morning and symmetrical joint pain (pain in the same joints on the two sides of the body) are the two hallmark symptoms of this disease. Tell your doctor all of your symptoms, even if they seem minor or you do not think they are important. Try to write down the answers to the following questions before you see the doctor:

- Where does it hurt?

- When does it hurt?

- When did it first begin to hurt?

- How long has it hurt?

- Have you any swelling?

- What daily tasks are difficult for you to do?

- Have you ever hurt the joint in an accident or overused it on the job or in a hobby?

- Has anyone in your family had similar problems?

The doctor will take X rays to look for damage to the joints and loss of minerals in the bones. Many doctors will X-ray both hands, to look for symmetrical damage to the joints—like the pain associated with rheumatoid arthritis, the joint damage will be symmetrical if you have the disease. Symmetrical damage to the joints, in addition to symmetrical pain and morning stiffness, almost certainly equals rheumatoid arthritis.

Aren't CT and MRI scans more accurate than X rays?

For diagnosing rheumatoid arthritis, an X ray is the best test, and early in the course of the disease the doctor probably will not do computed tomography (CT) or magnetic resonance imaging (MRI) scans. An MRI can be useful, however, in looking for problems in the spine in people with long-standing disease. For example, Marcie had confirmed rheumatoid arthritis for 20 years when she began experiencing neck pain and clicking in the joints when she moved her head. An MRI scan revealed a dislocation in her spine, which was fixed by fusing two vertebrae together, a simple procedure that prevented further damage. In another case, Jeffrey began having trouble moving his right leg after having rheumatoid arthritis for over 15 years. His doctor performed an MRI scan and found it was not involvement of the spine. Further tests revealed the problem to be a side effect of cortisone treatment. The problem cleared up when his cortisone dosage was decreased.

Isn't there something in the blood of people with rheumatoid arthritis?

Many, but not all, people with rheumatoid arthritis have an abnormal substance in their blood called rheumatoid factor. The doctor will test for this; it is not a specific test but it can help in the diagnosis—if you have it, you have a good chance of having rheumatoid arthritis, but if you don't, it doesn't mean you do not have the disease. About one quarter of people with rheumatoid arthritis do not have rheumatoid factor in their blood. People who do have rheumatoid factor, however, may develop worse disease than those who don't: Those who have rheumatoid factor have a 70% probability of developing joint damage or erosions within two years after the disease begins.

What other lab tests might my doctor perform?

The doctor may do an erythrocyte sedimentation rate (ESR), which is a measure of how fast your red blood cells settle after being mixed up. The ESR is a nonspecific measure of inflammation, and cannot distinguish between rheumatoid arthritis and other chronic inflammatory diseases, but it is a useful measure of the degree of inflammation. A decrease in the ESR indicates that your medication has been effective.

Blood tests may also indicate that you have anemia, which is common in chronic inflammatory diseases, and should decrease as your medication takes effect. Anemia can also be caused by long-term use of NSAIDs, including aspirin, which can irritate the lining of the stomach and cause bleeding. It is important for your doctor to tell which type of anemia you have, so you can be treated appropriately.

Your doctor might also perform tests on your blood to see how well your liver is working. People with rheumatoid arthritis often have minor changes in the functioning of their liver, because of the chronic inflammation caused by the disease. There is rarely any serious problem, however.

You might be asked to give a urine specimen to see how well your kidneys are working. Rheumatoid arthritis rarely affects the kidneys, but some of the medications you might be taking can.

My joints are so painful and swollen. Will the examination make them worse?

Your doctor will examine your joints carefully to see if they are swollen, compare them to look for symmetry, and feel them to see if they are hot. None of this will hurt. He may take synovial fluid from the joints that are painful and swollen. It might sound like it would hurt to take the fluid out of the affected joints, but it is really a simple and painless procedure. First, your doctor will inject some local anesthetic, which might burn a little. Then, he will stick a needle into the joint, between the bones, and withdraw some of the fluid. It might hurt a little when the fluid is removed and the inflamed tissues are allowed to rub against each other. This pain is very temporary and will subside almost immediately when the needle is removed.

Your doctor can get a lot of information from examining the synovial fluid. It should be yellow or straw-colored. If it is cloudy, that indicates the presence of cells or crystals, and the fluid will be examined under a microscope for the cells to be counted. If there are only a few cells, you could have rheumatoid arthritis or some other inflammatory disease like gout. Cells vary in number, and decisions are made based on the clinical picture (for example, a fever that is high and persistent), the character of the joint fluids, and sometimes the actual chemical substances in the joint fluid. If there are many cells, you might have an infection in your joint, which should be treated with antibiotics. Infections can also be distinguished from arthritis because an infection usually affects only one joint, not symmetrical joints. Cells and crystals mixed together in the synovial fluid indicate gout. How thick, or viscous, the synovial fluid is can provide additional information. Thick, gooey synovial fluid is normal, and has good lubricating qualities. Thin, watery synovial fluid means that cells have destroyed the lubricating qualities of the fluid and indicates a long-standing inflammation.

Will my doctor be able to tell me right away if I have rheumatoid arthritis?

It is difficult for any doctor, even a specialist, to give a definite diagnosis of rheumatoid arthritis on the first visit. The symptoms of this disease can be subtle, and not everyone has the same symptoms. Unlike a disease such as diabetes, there is no clear test that says "you have rheumatoid arthritis," so your doctor relies on a combination of several tests, using his skill and experience to finally reach a precise diagnosis. The symptoms of rheumatoid arthritis are similar to those associated with several other diseases, and it may take several visits to the doctor before the diagnosis is confirmed.

The American College of Rheumatology criteria for the diagnosis of rheumatoid arthritis include the following:

1. Morning stiffness (lasting at least one hour)

2. Swelling of the tissue around three or more joints

3. Swelling of the tissue around joints in the hands (PIP joint, MCP joint, or wrist)

4. Symmetric swelling of the tissue around joints

5. Nodules under the skin

6. The presence of rheumatoid factor in the blood

7. Erosion and/or loss of bone in the hand or wrist joints, seen on X ray

For a diagnosis of rheumatoid arthritis, you must have at least four of the seven symptoms listed. In addition, your doctor must have seen all of symptoms 1 through 4 for at least six weeks.

What type of doctor should I see?

Start with your family doctor or primary care physician. Your doctor should perform a complete physical examination, X-ray both hands to look for symmetrical joint damage, draw blood to test for rheumatoid factor and anemia, and draw fluid from swollen joints to look for cells and/or crystals. In most cases, your doctor should have you start taking DMARDs to prevent progression of the disease and anti-inflammatory drugs to ease the pain and swelling (see Chapter 3, "Other Available Treatments for Rheumatoid Arthritis").

If your doctor is up to date on arthritis diagnosis or treatments, you should continue to see him. Because rheumatoid arthritis affects only 1 in every 100 people, however, your doctor may not have much experience with this disease. If you or your doctor feels that he cannot adequately oversee your treatment, ask to be referred to an arthritis specialist, called a rheumatologist. In many cases, your doctor will have to justify this referral to your HMO or insurance agency, but this should be readily covered by your plan. Your doctor, local Arthritis Foundation, or insurance provider can provide you with a list of arthritis specialists in your area.

How often should I see the doctor?

Your disease and your response to treatment should be monitored carefully by your primary-care physician or rheumatologist. If you respond well to the medicines the doctor prescribes, and your symptoms disappear (are in remission), then your doctor may want to see you only twice a year. You may have to give blood or urine samples more frequently than that, depending on the medicines you are taking. For example, some of the DMARDs can affect your blood cells, and you must periodically have your blood tested to make sure your blood cell counts are normal. If the symptoms of arthritis continue to flare up, your doctor will want to see you every couple of months (see Chapter 3, "Other Available Treatments for Rheumatoid Arthritis").

Are there other types of specialists that can help?

Yes. Your primary-care physician or rheumatologist might also refer you to several other types of specialists to help with different aspects of your care (see Chapter 8, "Living with Rheumatoid Arthritis"). For example, a visiting nurse might come to your home to help with activities of daily living. Regular visits to a physical or occupational therapist can help you learn how to protect your joints from further damage, maintain the range of motion in joints affected by disease, and get started on a good exercise program that will strengthen your muscles without making you too tired. If you or your family members are feeling stressed or depressed about your condition, periodic visits with a social worker or clinical psychologist may help. If the arthritis is affecting your feet, a podiatrist may be able to offer some techniques to minimize the stress on those joints. Finally, if the disease is very advanced, you might consult with an orthopedic surgeon about having the joints operated on.

What types of surgery are performed on patients with rheumatoid arthritis?

As scary as surgery seems, most people who undergo some type of surgical procedure for rheumatoid arthritis are very happy with the results. And some of the procedures performed on people with rheumatoid arthritis are quite simple and relatively painless (see Chapter 3,

"Other Available Treatments for Rheumatoid Arthritis").

For example, arthroscopic surgery is performed under local anesthesia while you are awake and does not require an overnight stay in the hospital. The doctor will make a small incision near the joint and insert the tools through the incision to remove inflamed or damaged tissue. Once the procedure is done, all you will need is an adhesive bandage to cover the incision! And you will not be in bed for long—you should be walking again within one or two days.

In some cases, the surgeon can reduce the deformity in a joint by realigning or rebuilding the joint, which is more involved than arthroscopy and requires general anesthesia and a one- to two-week stay in the hospital.

If your joints are severely damaged, they may have to be replaced, using a technique called arthroplasty. The doctor will open up the joint, scrape off the heads of the bones that meet in the joint, and cap each bone with a metal or plastic head. The two caps are then joined by a spacer that acts as a hinge. Arthroplasty is performed most often on hips, knees, and hands. After arthroplasty you will probably have to have physical therapy to learn how to function the best way with your new joint.

TWO

What Are COX-2 Inhibitors?

- COX-2 inhibitors are a new class of drugs designed to relieve the pain associated with arthritis and related diseases.

- COX-2 inhibitors are one type of nonsteroidal anti-inflammatory drug (NSAID) but are more specific in their actions than are the other NSAIDs such as aspirin, ibuprofen, and naproxen (the COX-1 inhibitors).

- NSAIDs such as aspirin, ibuprofen, and naproxen are currently the most commonly used drugs to treat arthritis, and they are effective against the pain and swelling in this disease, but they also cause some side effects.

- The most common side effects of long-term use of NSAIDs are stomach pain and kidney failure. COX-2 inhibitors do not appear to have those side effects.

- About 19 million people in the United States take NSAIDs for their pain. Of those people, 76,000 develop ulcers that require them to go to the hospital, and 16,000 die each year from their ulcers. Doctors are excited about using COX-2 inhibitors to treat pain and swelling because they do not appear to have the serious side effects that current NSAIDs do.

What do you do? Your arthritis is acting up, your fingers are so sore and swollen that you can hardly move them. Your hip hurts no matter what position you're in. You are crabby and your coworkers are trying to be very careful around you so they don't set you off. You reach for the bottle of ibuprofen, which you know will relieve the pain somewhat, at least so you can finish up on the computer and go home. Then the sharp, stabbing pain begins again in your stomach, reminding you why you didn't take the ibuprofen earlier. It's your ulcer, caused by years of taking ibuprofen every day so you could function with your arthritis. What do you do? Live with the painful joints or aggravate the ulcer? It's not much of a choice.

Now you have another option! A brand-new type of drug, called the COX-2 inhibitor, acts just like the older NSAIDs to relieve the pain and swelling of rheumatoid arthritis, but does not cause ulcers! It won't cure your disease, but it sure will make it easier to live with.

∾ CASE STUDY

Herb is just 24 years old and has been playing football for the last 10 years. He played in high school and has been playing as a tight end for his college team. He recently developed back pain that made him seek medical attention. When seeing his doctor, he complained,

"I must have pulled a disk out of whack when I was playing football!"

While the doctor was performing a complete physical examination, Herb complained of pain in the right buttock and right lumbar region of his back. Asked how long it had been hurting, Herb replied that he'd been feeling pretty constant pain for about two weeks, but that it had been getting worse over the last few days, and that day it had really gotten bad. Herb told his doctor that the pain was particularly bad in the morning and typically got better as the day went on.

Herb had been taking Tylenol (acetaminophen) before going to bed, but was waking up at two or three o'clock in the morning with severe pain in his buttock and back, and could not get back to sleep. He then started taking aspirin for the pain, and he always took a couple before bed, which helped him sleep better and longer. He had recently started feeling very strong pains in his stomach on some mornings after taking aspirin.

When asked about previous bouts of pain in his back and buttock, Herb said that he suspected that he had had a slipped disk for years because he had "lumbago" when he was 20 years old, which caused pain in the left buttock. At that time, Herb took hot showers for the pain and found that sleeping with a heating pad made him feel better.

Herb's doctor asked about Herb's family history of medical problems. There was no history of arthritis in the family, but one of Herb's paternal aunts had psoriasis, as did Herb's father. On clinical examination, the doctor noted that Herb had pitted fingernails and some scaly skin under both armpits. Herb also had limited back movement and when the doctor performed some manipulations such as pressing on both hips to put pressure on the pelvis, the pain in the right buttock increased in intensity. The doctor told Herb that this meant that the pain was coming from a region of the back called the sacroiliac. The doctor diagnosed Herb with psoriatic arthritis.

Herb's pain was well controlled with a strong NSAID, but Herb had to take misoprostol, a synthetic prostaglandin, because of his stomach problems. The misoprostol gave Herb severe diarrhea, so he then tried the proton pump inhibitor Prilosec (omeprazole). The pain is now under control, but Herb still has problems with his stomach, and he is not sure how long he will be able to continue taking the NSAID. Herb and his doctor are eagerly awaiting the advent of COX-2 inhibitors, which will provide Herb with adequate pain relief without the danger of developing a stomach ulcer.

Herb's doctor recommended that Herb consult with a physical therapist. It will be difficult for someone as active as Herb to stop playing football, but the doctor assured him that the physical therapist will help him decide on a good exercise program that will help keep him fit.

How do COX-2 inhibitors work?

COX-2 inhibitors are NSAIDs just like the COX-1 inhibitors. (However, in this book, we will use the term NSAID to mean COX-1 inhibitors, to distinguish them from the new COX-2 inhibitors.) Both types of drug prevent the body from making a chemical called prostaglandin, and both do this by acting on enzymes called cyclooxygenases (COX). Researchers recently discovered that there are two forms of COX. One form, called COX 1, is made by cells all the time, and helps the body make prostaglandins that protect the stomach and regulate blood flow to the kidneys. The second form, COX

2, is made by the body mainly during inflammation, and is involved in the swelling and, indirectly, the pain associated with arthritis.

Traditional NSAIDs affect both COX 1 and COX 2, preventing the formation of both the ''good'' and ''bad'' prostaglandins. The decrease in the amount of good prostaglandin in the stomach may be why NSAIDs cause stomach pain. The good prostaglandins protect the stomach lining by increasing blood flow to that tissue and by helping to buffer the acidity in the stomach. These kinds of prostaglandins are sometimes called ''housekeeping'' prostaglandins, because they are involved in normal body functions. The best kind of NSAID would be one that does not destroy the prostaglandins involved in housekeeping chores within the body.

COX-2 inhibitors affect only COX 2, preventing the formation of the prostaglandins associated with inflammation, and not affecting the prostaglandins in the stomach and kidneys. Researchers and doctors hope that these drugs will provide relief for people with arthritis without causing stomach pain or ulcers or interfering with how the kidneys work.

Is COX 2 really only made during inflammation?

COX 2 is made in much larger amounts during inflammation than during normal cellular activities, but it is present in very low levels in some cells all the time. As researchers learn more about the functions of COX 2 in normal cells, we will also learn more about the possible long-term effects of taking these medicines. Right now, however, it appears that the COX-2 inhibitors mainly decrease pain and inflammation—positive effects—with very few, if any, negative effects.

In what tissues or organs is COX 2 normally found?

COX 2 is normally found in low levels in the brain, spinal cord, kidneys, pancreas, lungs, and stomach. Exactly what COX 2 is doing in these tissues is not known, but it is being studied by researchers. So far, no one has come up with a definite beneficial role for COX 2.

Some evidence suggests that in the kidney, COX 2 may regulate the concentration of salt in the urine and have an effect on blood pressure. COX 2 may also play a role in the development of the kidneys in the fetus. It is possible that COX 2 may be involved in the regulation of insulin secretion in the pancreas, and that too much COX 2 may be involved in type 2 diabetes. COX 2 is also found in the lungs, and it may have a role in the functioning of the blood vessels in the lungs. COX 2 may even be useful in healing gastric ulcers and may be important in preventing further damage in colitis.

COX 2 may also be required for the regulation and timing of events in early pregnancy. Levels of COX 2 increase during ovulation, the release of the egg from the ovary into the fallopian tube, where it can be fertilized. Even after ovulation, COX 2 is necessary for the successful implantation of the fertilized egg in the uterus. And finally, when it is time for the baby to be born, COX 2 is important in producing the prostaglandins that help the uterus contract. Some researchers are investigating a possible use for COX-2 inhibitors in preventing preterm labor (see Chapter 6, "Beyond Rheumatoid Arthritis: Other Uses for COX-2 Inhibitors").

Other possible roles for COX 2 in the normal functions of cells and tissues include bone remodeling and brain development in the fetus, but little is known about this enzyme in processes other than inflammation. Be assured, however, that research is going on and soon we will hear more about the other functions of COX 2 and possible uses for, and side effects of, COX-2 inhibitors.

When can I expect results with COX-2 inhibitors?

Like NSAIDs, a COX-2 inhibitor should work within an hour after taking the pill. With celecoxib (Celebrex), the first COX-2 inhibitor approved by the FDA (see page 49), the pain-relieving action lasts up to 12 hours, which means you will not have to remember to keep taking pills during the day, just one at breakfast and one after dinner. Rofecoxib (Vioxx) is also availible and has a specific indication for pain and is only taken once per day. While Vioxx does not have an indication for rheumatoid arthritis, it has the same anti-inflamatory effect as Celebrex.

Will COX-2 inhibitors cure my arthritis?

No. COX-2 inhibitors, like NSAIDs or corticosteroids, will not cure arthritis, but they will help alleviate the pain and swelling associated with the disease. COX-2 inhibitors are safer to use than NSAIDs or corticosteroids, because they do not produce the side effects of these other drugs.

Drugs of another type, called disease-modifying antirheumatic drugs, or DMARDs, can be taken to slow the progression of the disease (see Chapter 3, "Other Available Treatments for Rheumatoid Arthritis"). DMARDs comprise a wide variety of drugs, including hydroxychloroquine, gold salts, sulfasalazine, methotrexate, penicillamine, azathioprine, cyclophosphamide, cyclosporine, and leflunomide.

Your doctor will decide when it is appropriate for you to begin taking a DMARD and which one is best for you based on your symptoms, the cost and convenience of taking the drug, and the side effects of the drug. These are very powerful drugs and can cause some side effects, but most patients are happy to put up with the minor discomfort in exchange for slowing down the progression of the disease.

Ask your doctor about a combination of COX-2 inhibitors and DMARDs for the most effective treatment of arthritis. Effective pain relief with a COX-2 inhibitor can mask the fact that the disease process is still going on in the body, so it is important to take DMARDs as well as NSAIDs or COX-2 inhibitors, even if your joints are not too painful, to prevent further damage to the joints. Do not stop taking your DMARD when you start taking the COX-2 inhibitor.

Should I stop taking ibuprofen as soon as I start taking the COX-2 inhibitor?

Yes, you should stop taking any NSAID when you start taking the COX-2 inhibitor—you won't need the NSAID anymore! You can start taking the COX-2 inhibitor right away, and you shouldn't have any increase in pain during the switchover.

It is not a good idea to take more than one type of NSAID at a time, because the side effects of the NSAIDs might get worse if you take them together, and you should not take an NSAID with your COX-2 inhibitor either. Although the COX-2 inhibitors have a much better side effect profile than do other NSAIDs, they are not without side effects, and their long-term effects are still being investigated. So, to be safe, stop taking your NSAID and let the COX-2 inhibitor take over!

What about the other drugs I'm currently taking, like my DMARD? Can I continue taking that while I'm taking the COX-2 inhibitor?

By all means continue your DMARD therapy. COX-2 inhibitors do not replace DMARDs, and researchers have studied the effects of taking DMARDs and COX-2 inhibitors together, to make sure it is safe. In one study, patients took Celebrex and methotrexate together, and neither drug affected how the other worked, which means it is safe to take them together. There is some elevation of methotrexate blood levels when Vioxx is taken at the same time as methotrexate, so caution is warranted if you are on both of these drugs.

Researchers have also found that caution must be used when Celebrex or Vioxx is given with warfarin, a drug to prevent blood clots. Recent data have shown that both Celebrex and Vioxx increase the effects of warfarin, resulting in an increased thinning of the blood, but this increase is thought to be insignificant.

Researchers have also found that Celebrex and warfarin, a drug to prevent blood clots, do not affect each other. This is exceptionally good news, since prior to this time NSAIDs could never be taken with a blood thinner. Caution is needed, however, since some bleeding has occurred with Celebrex, but it is not clear if the bleeding was caused by Celebrex.

More information on drug interactions is available in the package insert that comes with the COX-2 inhibitor, so be sure to read that. Also, tell your doctor about all the drugs you are taking, even ones you think are perfectly safe, to make sure that your COX-2 inhibitor will not interfere with those drugs, or vice versa.

Can I stop taking corticosteroids?

Do not stop taking corticosteroids without talking to your doctor. He might decide that it is all right for you to stop taking corticosteroids and to just rely on the COX-2 inhibitor, with an occasional injection of corticosteroid if a particular joint flares up. But you should not stop or start any medication without talking to your doctor first. It is especially important not to stop taking corticosteroids suddenly because you might experience a flare-up of the symptoms. You need to start by tapering the dose, so that you give your body time to start making its own corticosteroids.

How long have COX-2 inhibitors been around?

COX-2 inhibitors were discovered by researchers in 1990, and several pharmaceutical companies are now working on the final stages of development of their products and awaiting FDA approval. Two COX-2 inhibitors, Celebrex and Vioxx, have been approved for use by the FDA and are available by prescription. Vioxx is particularly efficient, and is expected to be a very selective COX-2 inhibitor. Also in development, meloxicam is an NSAID that inhibits COX-2 much more than COX-1, but still has some activity against COX-1. It's called a preferential COX-2 inhibitor rather than a selective COX-2 inhibitor.

These drugs have been tested in extensive clinical trials involving thousands of people with arthritis, both rheumatoid arthritis and osteoarthritis (see Chapter 4, "Are COX-2 Inhibitors Safe and Effective?"). The results of testing Celebrex, Vioxx, and meloxicam have been made public and demonstrate clearly that these drugs work as well as traditional NSAIDs, but do not cause nearly as many ulcers. People taking Celebrex at doses of 100 mg or 200 mg twice a day had as much pain relief as those taking naproxen 500 mg twice a day, but did not get any ulcers. One quarter of the people taking naproxen got ulcers. A meloxicam dose of 7.5 mg or 15 mg was also as good as naproxen or piroxicam (Feldene) at relieving the pain associated with rheumatoid arthritis, while causing far fewer ulcers. Another study compared Vioxx at 250 mg/day with aspirin at 650 mg four times a day and ibuprofen at 600 mg three times a day. (Vioxx is actually effective at a much lower dose of 12.5 or 25 mg a day.) People in this study who were taking Vioxx had problems with their stomachs roughly as often as those taking only a sugar pill, while almost all of the people taking aspirin and three quarters of those taking ibuprofen had problems. (See Chapter 4, "Are COX-2 Inhibitors Safe and Effective?" for more details.)

Are there different kinds of COX-2 inhibitors?

There are at least seven different COX-2 inhibitors currently in development. Although these products all have different chemical structures, they all act by inhibiting the enzyme COX-2.

Celebrex, manufactured by Searle, a subdivision of Monsanto, was approved by the FDA at the end of 1998 and Vioxx, manufactured by Merck & Co., became available in 1999. Meloxicam, manufactured by Boehringer Ingelheim, is still being tested in clinical trials in the United States, but has been available in other countries under the names Mobic, Mobec, Movalis, Movatec, and Mobicox. Roche Laboratories, Johnson & Johnson, and Glaxo Wellcome PLC also have COX-2 inhibitors in development.

All of the COX-2 inhibitors cause very few side effects such as stomach pain and kidney disease. In fact, in one clinical trial, people taking the COX-2 inhibitor Celebrex for one week experienced no ulcers, while 6 of the 32 people taking naproxen for one week did get ulcers. Meloxicam has also been extensively tested in clinical trials. In these trials, people taking meloxicam experienced far fewer ulcers than did those taking naproxen or piroxicam (Feldene). People taking naproxen also had more problems with their kidneys. In a study comparing Vioxx with aspirin and ibuprofen, both aspirin and ibuprofen caused far more ulcers than did Vioxx. (See Chapter 4, "Are COX-2 Inhibitors Safe and Effective?" for more details.)

How do I know which COX-2 inhibitor to take?

At the beginning you will not have much choice, because only two COX-2 inhibitors, Celebrex and Vioxx, are available. When more are available, your doctor will help you decide which is the best for you.

Once you have started taking a COX-2 inhibitor that works for you, there is no reason to change. If, however, you find that the drug is not relieving the pain and swelling you experience, talk to your doctor about switching to a different COX-2 inhibitor. Since the drugs are all different chemically, one may work better than another for you. Switching should not be a problem—these medicines do not stay in your body very long and no withdrawal effects have been noticed when people have stopped taking them.

Can COX-2 inhibitors help with the symptoms of other types of arthritis?

Yes, these medicines are expected to treat not just rheumatoid arthritis, but many other types of arthritis as well. Celebrex has been tested in a clinical trial of 1,004 people with osteoarthritis who were experiencing painful flare-ups. As it did in people with rheumatoid arthritis, Celebrex worked as well as naproxen at relieving the pain of osteoarthritis and caused fewer side effects. Vioxx is particularly effective in the relief of osteoarthritis pain, menstrual pain, and pain from sports injuries.

COX-2 inhibitors will be used to alleviate the pain caused by many of the arthritis-like diseases, and will probably also be used for headaches, menstrual pain, and sports injuries as well—in fact for any problem that is now treated with aspirin, ibuprofen, or naproxen (see Chapter 6, "Beyond Rheumatoid Arthritis: Other Uses for COX-2 Inhibitors," for more information).

Will I be able to take a COX-2 inhibitor if I am pregnant?

We don't know yet, but at this time the answer is a definite no! The results of studies on how COX-2 inhibitors affect pregnant women or fetuses have not yet been made public. However, as mentioned on page 121, preterm labor may be able to be eliminated with COX-2 inhibitors because the COX-2 enzyme is involved in the formation of the prostaglandins that help the uterus contract and expel the baby into the world. As with any medication, before taking a COX-2 inhibitor, speak to your doctor if you are thinking about getting pregnant, or are already pregnant and plan to take a COX-2 inhibitor. This is because early studies in mice indicated that such inhibitors caused some degree of infertility when the mice were given the drug while pregnancy was attempted. Until it is clear that it is safe to take COX-2 inhibitors while pregnant, do not take chances; if you are taking COX-2 inhibitors, either use a reliable method of birth control or stop taking the medicine. If you are already pregnant, do not start taking COX-2 inhibitors until more is known about their effects during pregnancy.

I'm still breastfeeding our baby and I'd like to try a COX-2 inhibitor. Is this safe?

We do not know if COX-2 inhibitors are safe to take while breastfeeding, and this is a decision that needs to be made based on the severity of your illness. Since there is a certain degree of COX-2 inhibition with traditional NSAIDs, it is unlikely that the COX-2 inhibitors will have a detrimental effect in mother's milk. No information, however, on whether or not COX-2 inhibitors are excreted through breast milk has been made available, so it is best to wait until you stop breastfeeding before starting the COX-2 inhibitor because all elective drugs (medications not essential for survival) should be eliminated during the nursing period. However, if you are already taking a COX-2 inhibitor, the chances are that they will be quite safe to the baby and, most importantly, will allow you to function in the care of your new infant. Consult your doctor regarding taking or continuing to take this medication while breastfeeding.

THREE

Other Available Treatments for Rheumatoid Arthritis

- Nonsteroidal anti-inflammatory drugs (NSAIDs)

- Salicylates

- Corticosteroids

- Analgesics

- Disease-modifying antirheumatic drugs (DMARDs)

✿ CASE STUDY

Mary, a 58-year-old insurance sales agent, had had rheumatoid arthritis for 25 years. Mary had well-established disease, with severe pain in her neck. She was unable to flex her neck—she could move it only about 40% as much as she could 10 years before—and when she did move her head, pain radiated behind her ear. She was no longer able to function at work or even to do basic household chores, so she decided to talk to her doctor about surgery.

The doctor performed a complete physical exam and went over Mary's history carefully. She noted that Mary was unable to produce tears readily and had had dry mouth for about three years. The joints in both of Mary's hands were destroyed, with swellings in the wrists and in several small finger joints, elbows, and ankles. Mary had rheumatoid factor in her blood and a sedimentation rate of 60. X rays of Mary's neck showed that the odontoid bone (one of the bones in the spine) was eroded and that the atlas bone (the first vertebra in the neck) was significantly displaced, which might eventually result in paralysis.

Mary's doctor immediately scheduled her for cervical spine surgery to stabilize her neck. In the meantime, she instructed Mary to wear a cervical collar.

Mary had been treated with sulfasalazine (Azulfidine) 2 grams per day taken in divided doses for the last five years and prednisone 20 mg per day for the past two years. She only took the prednisone when she had severe pain, which was roughly two weeks out of every month. Mary had also tried several NSAIDs, but none of them worked really well to relieve her pain. In the last year, Mary had tried taking codeine for the pain.

Mary's doctor started her on methotrexate (Rheumatrex) 2.5 mg three pills every week, for a weekly total of 7.5 mg. She explained to Mary that the dose would be increased later. Mary also started taking folic acid 1 mg per day to minimize the side effects of methotrexate. The doctor decided to taper the prednisone and eventually Mary would stop taking the corticosteroid. Mary's doctor discussed with her two new drugs that had recently been approved by the FDA, etanercept (Enbrel) and leflunomide (Arava). If Mary did not respond well to methotrexate, she would try one of the newer drugs.

The doctor added a mild analgesic, tramadol (Ultram), to a strict regimen of NSAID, which Mary would have to take with either misoprostil (synthetic prostaglandin) or a proton pump inhibitor such as omeprazole (Prilosec) to protect her from getting a stomach ulcer. A COX-2 inhibitor would be perfect for Mary, who needed strong pain control but had trouble with stomach pain when she took an NSAID.

What are the traditional treatments for rheumatoid arthritis?

Anti-inflammatory drugs, like aspirin, ibuprofen, or naproxen sodium (NSAIDs), can help relieve joint swelling, stiffness, and pain. The NSAIDs are listed in Table 3. NSAIDs work by preventing the body from making a type of chemical called prostaglandins, which are involved in the swelling and, indirectly, the pain associated with arthritis. After taking an NSAID you should feel pain relief within an hour, but you may not notice the swelling going down until you have been taking the drug regularly for a week or two.

NSAIDs act on an enzyme called cyclooxygenase (COX), which exists in two forms, COX 1 and COX 2. COX 1 is used by all cells to help the body make prostaglandins that have "housekeeping" functions, particularly in the stomach and kidneys. These prostaglandins help protect the stomach from getting ulcers and regulate blood flow to the kidneys. COX 2 is used to make a different type of prostaglandins, only made during inflammation, which cause the pain and swelling associated with inflammation in rheumatoid arthritis and other diseases. (See Chapter 2, "What Are COX-2 Inhibitors?" for a discussion of the differences between these traditional NSAIDs and COX-2 inhibitors, a newer form of NSAID.)

Unfortunately, traditional NSAIDs cannot distinguish between the two types of COX enzymes, and they inhibit both. Long-term use of NSAIDs such as ibuprofen or aspirin can cause stomach ulcers because of their action on COX 1. Some types of NSAID act on COX 1 more than others, which may cause them to cause more ulcers.

Do all NSAIDs inhibit COX 1 and COX 2 to the same degree?

No. The NSAIDs vary in the degree to which they inhibit COX 1 and COX 2, and this may be one reason why some NSAIDs are better tolerated than others. Drugs that inhibit COX 2 to a much greater extent than COX 1 may cause fewer ulcers.

Meloxicam is called a preferential COX-2 inhibitor, as opposed to the selective COX-2 inhibitors described in Chapter 2, because it inhibits COX 2 ten to 100 times as much as it does COX 1, but still has significant activity against COX 1. Because it does inhibit COX 2 more, however, meloxicam causes far fewer stomach problems than do other NSAIDs. Meloxicam has been compared with piroxicam and naproxen in people with rheumatoid arthritis, and was found to be as effective at relieving the pain of arthritis as the other NSAIDs while causing far fewer ulcers. Similar results were obtained in people with osteoarthritis, comparing meloxicam with piroxicam and diclofenac (see Chapter 4, "Are COX-2 Inhibitors Safe and Effective?" for more details). Meloxicam was also shown to be safe in people with arthritis who had moderate kidney problems.

Table 3. NSAIDs

Drug*	Common Brand Name(s)	Dosage**
Diclofenac potassium	Cataflam	75 to 100 mg/day in a single dose
Diclofenac sodium	Voltaren	100 to 150 mg/day in 2 doses
Etodolac	Lodine	400 to 1,200 mg/day in 1 to 4 doses
Fenoprofen calcium	Nalfon	900 to 2,400 mg/day in 3 or 4 doses; never more than 3,200 mg/day
Flurbiprofen sodium	Ansaid	200 to 300 mg/day in 2 or 3 doses
Ibuprofen	Motrin, Motrin IB, Advil, Nuprin (other brands also available)	1,200 to 3,200 mg/day in 3 or 4 doses
Indomethacin	Indocin	50 to 200 mg/day in 2 to 4 doses

---

*Nonacetylated salicylates, drugs related to aspirin, are listed in Table 5. **The exact dosage will be determined by your doctor, taking into account the severity of your condition, your age, and your weight.

Ketoprofen	Orudis, Orudis KT, Oruvail, Actron	150 to 300 mg/day in 3 or 4 doses
Ketorolac tromethamine	Toradol	Oral: Up to 40 mg/day in 4 to 6 doses Injected: Up to 120 mg/day in 4 doses
Meclofenamate sodium	Meclomen	200 to 400 mg/day in 3 or 4 doses
Mefenamic acid	Ponstel	1,000 mg/day in 4 doses
Nabumetone	Relafen	500 to 1,500 mg/day in 2 or 3 doses
Naproxen	Naprosyn	500 to 1500 mg/day in 2 or 3 doses
Naproxen sodium	Anaprox, Aleve	550 to 1650 mg/day in 2 or 3 doses
Oxaprozin	Daypro	1,200 to 1,800 mg/day in a single dose
Piroxicam	Feldene	20 mg/day in a single dose
Sulindac	Clinoril	300 to 400 mg/day in 2 doses
Tolmetin sodium	Tolectin	1,200 to 1,800 mg/day in 3 doses

Do NSAIDs act only on COX 1 and COX 2, or are there other systems involved?

The biological systems involved in inflammation are very complex, and it would be too simple if only COX enzymes were affected by NSAIDs. So, the answer is, many other systems are probably affected by NSAIDs, and researchers are beginning to figure out which ones and how. Part of the reason for figuring out which systems are affected is to try to develop drugs that work more specifically on pain and inflammation, without causing as many side effects. The selective COX-2 inhibitors are a good start on this effort (see Chapter 2, "What Are COX-2 Inhibitors?").

Cytokines are molecules produced by cells during inflammation, which can aggravate the inflammation by recruiting more immune cells. There is some evidence that NSAIDs such as meloxicam, piroxicam, indomethacin, and diclofenac may inhibit some cytokines, thereby decreasing inflammation by both their effect on COX enzymes and their inhibition of cytokine production. NSAIDs may also have a direct effect on some white blood cells, called neutrophils, involved in inflammation.

Another pathway for inflammation is called the nitric oxide pathway. Nitric oxide is produced by an enzyme called nitric oxide synthase and has effects similar to prostaglandins, that is, in small amounts it may help protect the stomach lining and in larger amounts it enhances the inflammatory response. Increased levels of nitric oxide and other products of this pathway have been found in the synovial fluid of people with rheumatoid arthritis. These chemicals may be involved in the degradation of cartilage that occurs in the joints. Researchers have shown that some NSAIDs can inhibit the production of nitric oxide, independent of their effect on COX 1 or

COX 2. Understanding this pathway has started researchers developing more specific drugs, called nitro-NSAIDs, which are NSAIDs coupled to a nitric oxide–releasing compound, which may provide better protection of the stomach lining (see Chapter 7, "The Future of Rheumatoid Arthritis Treatment").

Do all NSAIDs cause the same side effects?

NSAIDs do cause all the same types of side effects, but they differ widely in the extent of those side effects. Several research groups have investigated and compared the side effects of different NSAIDs, and have found that some NSAIDs are as much as four times more likely to cause side effects than others. NSAIDs can be ranked according to their tendency to cause stomach ulcers (Table 4). Your doctor will help you choose the best NSAID for you. You might not have a problem with ulcers or other side effects, and you may find that one drug works better for you than another.

How can I reduce my chances of getting an ulcer while taking an NSAID?

To reduce the chances of getting an ulcer, take the NSAID with food rather than on an empty stomach. If you already have stomach pain from taking NSAIDs, three types of drug are available that might help. The first is a class called histamine blockers, or H_2 blockers, which reduce the amount of acid produced by the stomach. Histamine blockers include cimetidine (Tagamet), ranitidine hydrochloride (Zantac), famotidine (Pepcid), and nizatidine (Axid). The second class is the proton pump inhibitors, including omeprazole (Prilosec) and lansoprazole (Prevacid). You should be careful when

Table 4. NSAID Gastrointestinal Toxicity Ranking*

NSAID**	Toxicity Rank
Salsalate (related to aspirin, see page 69)	1
Aspirin	2
Ibuprofen	3
Sulindac	4
Naproxen	5
Piroxicam	6
Tolmetin sodium	7
Diclofenac	8
Indomethacin	9
Fenoprofen calcium	10
Ketoprofen	11
Meclofenamate sodium	12

*A score of 1 is least toxic.
**Not all of the medicines listed in Table 3 are listed here.

taking histamine blockers or antacids, because these drugs may make you feel better while the ulcer is still there. The third class consists of only one drug, misoprostol (Cytotec), which is a synthetic prostaglandin. This drug works by replacing the prostaglandins that protect your stomach, reducing the chances of developing an ulcer and helping to heal existing ulcers. Misoprostol is expensive, however, and can cause diarrhea, but it can be very helpful in people who require a particular NSAID for pain relief. A combination of diclofenac and misoprostol, called Arthrotec, is now available (see Chapter 7, "The Future of Rheumatoid Arthritis Treatment").

Some of the anti-ulcer medications are available over the counter (OTC), but to be safe, you should talk to your doctor before selecting an anti-ulcer medicine about whether one of these drugs might be good for you.

I can just get ibuprofen or aspirin at the drug store. Why do I need to see a doctor?

Many NSAIDs are available OTC or by prescription. NSAIDs can be taken orally, and some are available by injection or as rectal suppositories for people who have trouble taking medication orally. When taken over a long period of time, NSAIDs can cause stomach ulcers, so be sure to consult your doctor, even when using OTC medicines. It is also important to see a doctor because there are other medicines that you might need to help control the symptoms of rheumatoid arthritis and possibly slow the progression of the disease.

Even though NSAIDs are available OTC, they can cause problems and should be used very carefully. Seniors, people with diseases such as hypertension, diabetes, congestive heart failure, kidney damage, or cirrhosis (liver damage), and people taking other medicines that affect the kidneys can take NSAIDs but must be carefully watched to make sure there is no damage to the kidneys.

Some NSAIDs, such as ibuprofen and aspirin, can be taken by children and are available in lower dosage tablets and liquid specifically for children.

Aspirin and ibuprofen should not be taken by pregnant women or nursing mothers, because there might be a chance of damage to the fetus or infant. Fortunately, some evidence exists that the symptoms of rheumatoid arthritis diminish during pregnancy, and you may find it is not necessary to take an NSAID during this time. If the pain and swelling persist, ask your doctor about other medications you might take.

Is the risk of getting a stomach ulcer really that high for people taking NSAIDs?

Yes, and there is a lot of evidence to support this statement. A very large study was conducted on people taking NSAIDs for rheumatoid arthritis and other diseases, called the ARAMIS study. More than 24,000 people were contacted to fill out a questionnaire about their use of NSAIDs and the side effects they experienced. One of the first things that became obvious was that there is a definite problem with stomach ulcers in patients taking NSAIDs.

The researchers then focused on the 2,747 people with rheumatoid arthritis included in the larger group. They found that people taking NSAIDs were five times as likely to be hospitalized, and twice as likely to die because of stomach problems as were people not taking NSAIDs. Seniors, people taking prednisone as well as an NSAID, people who had previous stomach problems, and people who were more disabled were at greatest risk for hospitalization and/or death. This study found that women were not at higher risk than men.

The researchers conducting the ARAMIS study estimated that 76,000 hospitalizations per year could be attributed to NSAID use, of which 26,000 hospitalizations were of patients with rheumatoid arthritis. They also estimated that 21% of the 76,000 died—that means that 16,000 deaths per year in all people who take NSAIDs, and 2,600 deaths of people with rheumatoid arthritis, are directly due to NSAID-induced ulcers.

These numbers for hospitalization and death are very high, and indicate that patients who take NSAIDs for a long time must be carefully watched. See your doctor regularly and let him know if you have any signs of ulcer, such as pain or indigestion.

The ARAMIS study sounds very useful. Is it still going on?

Yes, the ARAMIS 2000 survey is still going on, and the researchers are looking for more people with rheumatoid arthritis to join. The goal of this study is to improve long-term outcomes in arthritis by learning how arthritis affects people over time. This is not a drug trial; all that is required is for you to fill out a questionnaire that you will receive in the mail every six months. The questionnaire will ask questions about your pain, fatigue, physical functioning, mood, medicines, and medical care. All answers will be confidential, and the researchers will not ask you to change your medication in any way. If you participate in ARAMIS 2000, you will also receive a newsletter with each questionnaire. The newsletter will describe what projects are being conducted using the information from all the questionnaires, as well as other information of interest to people with rheumatoid arthritis. For more information, check out the Stanford University Department of Rheumatology website (www.stanford.edu/group/rheum/rheuhome.html), or call (650)723-5928. You may call collect if this is a long-distance call.

Can I take ibuprofen and aspirin together when the pain is really bad?

No, you should not take NSAIDs in combination with each other. This might make the side effects even worse, and it has not been proven that NSAIDs in combination work better than alone. If your pain is not getting better with the NSAID that your doctor prescribed, call your doctor and let him know. Your medication may need to be adjusted. You may need to take a stronger dose or a different NSAID, or your disease-modifying antirheumatic drug (DMARD) may need to be changed or the dosage adjusted. Do not do this on your own, however. Always call your doctor when your medication is not working.

Don't people take steroids for rheumatoid arthritis?

Yes, steroids are used in the treatment of rheumatoid arthritis—they have been used for almost 50 years to reduce inflammation in rheumatoid arthritis and other inflammatory diseases. Because they act quickly, these drugs are often used for a short time while waiting for DMARDs to work. The DMARDs actually slow the progression of the disease but take longer to work than do corticosteroids. Corticosteroids can also be taken during flare-ups, and then stopped when the flare-up has resolved.

Cortisone is a steroid hormone that is made in our bodies by glands called the adrenal glands. Cortisone and its relatives, such as dexamethasone, prednisone, and hydrocortisone, are in a class of drugs called corticosteroids. These drugs act one step before NSAIDs and the COX-2 inhibitors in the chain of events that lead to inflammation: Corticosteroids inhibit the activity of an enzyme called phospholipase A_2. Phospholipase A_2 causes the release of arachidonic acid, which is the chemical from which prostaglandin is made. Ultimately, then, corticosteroids have effects similar to those of NSAIDs and COX-2 inhibitors, but even broader effects, and side effects, because they act at an earlier step.

These drugs can be taken orally or by intravenous injection, to have a broad effect on your whole body. As well as having an anti-inflammatory effect, corticosteroids may also help to suppress the immune system, which is overactive in rheumatoid arthritis.

If only one or two joints are affected by the disease, your doctor may choose to inject the drug directly into the joint; when administered this way, the drug will act quickly and will not produce the side effects that taking it orally or by intravenous injection do.

What are the side effects caused by corticosteroids?

Corticosteroids can have serious side effects and are often taken daily or every other day in small doses; a larger dose can then be taken during a flare-up of symptoms. This strategy reduces the chances of side effects, such as weight gain, water retention, unusual fat distribution (which causes a characteristic puffy face called moon face and a deformity of the back called buffalo hump), thin skin, cataracts, high blood pressure, osteoporosis (thin, brittle bones), and mood changes.

Women who have already gone through menopause and are not taking hormone replacement therapy must be particularly careful when taking corticosteroids because there is a much greater risk of bone fracture once your body stops producing estrogen. Be sure to take adequate amounts of calcium and vitamin D. Talk to your doctor about taking a drug called calcitonin, which helps increase the strength of the bones. You might want to consider hormone replacement therapy, which supplies some of the estrogen your body stops making after menopause. If you have already experienced a significant amount of bone loss, consider taking drugs such as etidronate or alendronate, which can treat bone loss. Some types of diuretics, called thiazide diuretics, reduce the amount of calcium lost in urine. If you need to take a diuretic, ask your doctor if this might be useful.

You might be able to reduce the severity of the side effects by taking the following steps:

- To reduce swelling, try eliminating salt from your diet.

- Muscle wasting can be counteracted by increasing your exercise.

- Osteoporosis can be slowed by taking calcium and vitamin D supplements.

- Mood changes such as depression might be helped by high doses of vitamin C, psychotherapy, or low doses of an antidepressant.

If you find that the side effects are so unpleasant that you need to stop taking the corticosteroid, you might have to taper off your dosage slowly over a period of time, especially if you have been taking the corticosteroid for a long time. This is because taking additional amounts of a natural substance, such as a corticosteroid, can cause your body to shut down its own production and it will take awhile for the body to readjust and begin making its own cortisone again.

Talk to your doctor if you are thinking about getting

pregnant and are taking a corticosteroid. It is always better not to take drugs if you do not have to while you are pregnant or nursing. Corticosteroids can be taken by children, but can affect growth, so children should be carefully monitored and the dose should be kept as low as possible. You will also be more susceptible to infections while taking a corticosteroid.

I usually take acetaminophen for my headaches, because it's easier on my stomach than ibuprofen. Will that help with my arthritis?

Acetaminophen is a very effective pain reliever, but does not reduce inflammation. Thus it is not used often in rheumatoid arthritis, but it is often used in osteoarthritis. Acetaminophen can be used for pain relief and to reduce fever, however, and does not cause ulcers. Unlike the NSAIDs and COX-2 inhibitors, acetaminophen does not work by inhibiting the action of the enzyme COX. Rather, it acts on an area of the brain called the hypothalamic heat-regulating center to reduce fever, possibly by preventing prostaglandin production. Acetaminophen acts to reduce pain by acting directly on the pain threshold, again probably by preventing prostaglandin production.

Long-term use of acetaminophen may cause liver damage, especially if used with alcohol. Acetaminophen is safe for use by children, but should not be used by people with anemia or liver or kidney disease.

Acetaminophen is sometimes used in combination with a narcotic drug, such as codeine, and some doctors prescribe propoxyphene hydrochloride (Darvon) for the pain associated with arthritis. Be careful with narcotic drugs, however, as they can cause sleepiness—you

should not drive or perform tasks that require alertness—
and are addicting.

Can I just take aspirin?

Aspirin acts to block cyclooxygenase and prevent
prostaglandin production, so it helps relieve the pain and
swelling associated with rheumatoid arthritis, but it can
cause ulcers or internal bleeding. Even buffered or
enteric-coated aspirin (aspirin with a special coating to
make the medicine easier on your stomach) can cause
ulcers, although they are better than plain aspirin.

Many other related drugs are now available, and most
doctors do not recommend taking aspirin for rheumatoid
arthritis. For example, drugs related to aspirin, called
nonacetylated salicylates, are easier on the stomach and
can be taken less frequently than aspirin (Table 5). These
drugs also will not increase your tendency to bleed,
which aspirin can do. Nonacetylated salicylates are also
NSAIDs; talk with your doctor about which type of anti-
inflammatory drug might be best for you.

Aren't there creams that can help relieve the pain?

Yes, some creams or rubs, called topical analgesics,
can be used to relieve pain if it is mild and affects only
a few joints. You might also try a topical analgesic if
your oral NSAID or aspirin is not working, or if you are
unable to take an oral drug. The nice thing about topical
analgesics is that they have very little risk of causing
the side effects that oral drugs do.

Topical analgesics often contain salicylates, just like
aspirin. When you rub the cream into your skin, the
salicylate is absorbed into your tissues, where it prevents
the production of prostaglandins, just like aspirin that

Table 5. Nonacetylated Salicylates

Drug	Brand Name(s)	Dosage*
Choline magnesium trisalicylate	CMT, Tricosal, Trilisate	3,000 mg/day in 2 or 3 doses
Choline salicylate	Arthropan	3,480 to 6,960 mg/day in several doses
Diflunisal	Dolobid	500 to 1,000 mg/day in 2 doses
Magnesium salicylate	Magan, Doan's Pills, Mobidin	2,600 to 4,800 mg/day in 3 to 6 doses
Salsalate	Disalcid, Mono-Gesic, Salflex, Salsitab, Amigesic, Anaflex 750, Marthritic	1,500 to 3,000 mg/day in 2 or 3 doses
Sodium salicylate	(Available as generic only)	1,950 to 3,900 mg/day in several doses

*The exact dosage will be determined by your doctor, taking into account the severity of your condition, your age, and your weight.

you take orally. But the topical analgesics act locally, meaning that the salicylate does not travel far from where you rub it in, so you do not have to worry about ulcers. Some topical analgesics that contain salicylates include Aspercreme, BenGay, Flexall, Mobisyl, and Sportscreme.

Another way to help relieve the pain of arthritis is to distract your brain so that it does not notice your joints hurt. Many topical analgesics also contain substances called counterirritants, such as menthol, oil of wintergreen, camphor, eucalyptus oil, turpentine oil, dihydrochloride, and methylnicotinate. Counterirritants work by actually irritating the nerves around the joint—your brain will become so busy with that new sensation that it does not notice the more significant joint pain caused by the arthritis. Some products that act mainly as counterirritants include ArthriCare, Eucalyptamint, Icy Hot, and Therapeutic Mineral Ice.

The stuff that makes hot peppers hot, called capsaicin, can also help your joint pain. When you rub creams containing capsaicin on your joints, the nerves around the joint release less of a chemical called substance P (for pain). Substance P is one of the chemicals that sends the pain message to your brain, and if the nerves do not release it, your brain does not know about the pain. Zostrix, Zostrix HP, and Cazasin-P are some creams that contain capsaicin. Menthacin contains both capsaicin and counterirritants.

These products may seem safe to use because they are just creams, but you should still be very careful using them. Be sure to tell your doctor that you are, especially if you are allergic to aspirin. And don't forget, these products are just fooling the brain into forgetting about the real source of the pain; they are not treating the arthritis itself.

Are there any drugs that cure rheumatoid arthritis, or at least stop it from getting worse?

No drugs have yet been found that will cure rheumatoid arthritis, but DMARDs work to slow, and in some cases halt, the progression of the disease.

If you have had symptoms for three months or more; have been taking an NSAID; and still have joint pain, significant morning stiffness or fatigue, or inflammation, ask your doctor about taking a DMARD. Until recently, most doctors did not prescribe DMARDs until a patient's symptoms stopped responding to other therapies, such as NSAIDs or corticosteroids, but now doctors are treating rheumatoid arthritis much more aggressively and starting DMARD treatment earlier.

Starting treatment with DMARDs early in the course of the disease may prevent damage from accumulating, and may prevent your joints from being irreversibly damaged. The goal of early treatment with DMARDs is to intervene before joints are damaged. If you have had arthritis for a while, and have had X rays that show damage to the joints, you should start taking a DMARD immediately to prevent further damage.

DMARDs include hydroxychloroquine, gold salts, sulfasalazine, methotrexate, penicillamine, azathioprine, and cyclophosphamide (see Table 6).

How do I know which DMARD is the best to take?

There is no way of knowing which one will work best

Table 6. DMARDs

Drug	Brand Name (s)	Onset of Action	Response Rate	Dosage*
Azathioprine	Imuran	2–3 months	30%–50%	100–150 mg/day
Cyclophosphamide	Cytoxan	1–3 months	50%	2 mg/kg oral; 750–1,000 mg/m², IV
Cyclosporine	Sandimmune, Neoral	1–3 months	50%	2.5 mg/kg/day
Etanercept	Enbrel	1–2 weeks	40%–70%	25 mg subcutaneously twice weekly
Gold (injectable)	Myochrysine (gold sodium thiomalate), Solganal (aurothioglucose)	3–6 months	30%	50 mg/week
Gold (oral)	Ridaura (aurofin)	6 months	20%	3–9 mg/day
Hydroxychloroquine	Plaquenil	2–6 months	30%–50%	200 mg twice daily
Leflunomide	Arava	1–3 months	10%–40%	20 mg/day
Methotrexate	Rheumatrex	6–8 weeks	Greater than 70%	7.5–15 mg/week
Minocycline	Minocin, Dynacin	3–6 months	5%–30%	100 mg twice daily
D-penicillamine	Cuprimine, Depen	3–6 months	10%–30%	750–1,000 mg daily in divided doses
Sulfasalazine	Azulfidine	2–3 months	Greater than 30%	1 g 2 or 3 times/day

*The exact dosage will be determined by your doctor, taking into account the severity of your condition, your age, and your weight.

for you, but two thirds of patients have a good response to one or more DMARDs. The DMARDs are all very different types of drugs, and they act in different ways and have different side effects. Your doctor will discuss which might be best suited for you, taking into account the convenience of taking the drug (some are taken only once a day, while others are taken up to four times a day), the cost of the drug, whether any monitoring is necessary (and its cost), how long until you begin to feel the effects, and the side effects of each type of drug. Any other diseases, such as a heart condition or kidney or liver disease, that you might have will affect the choice of DMARD. In addition, the severity of your disease will help determine which DMARD to start with.

I've heard of patients taking an anti-malarial drug called hydroxychloroquine. Is that a good drug to start with?

Yes. Hydroxychloroquine (Plaquenil) is a good DMARD to start with for patients with mild to moderate disease. This drug has a good safety profile and can be taken once or twice a day, but it takes two to six months to work. Hydroxychloroquine seems to affect the function of immune system cells and is also used to treat malaria. Some of the side effects of this drug are diarrhea, loss of appetite, nausea, stomach cramps or pain, and black spots in your vision. This drug does not affect your blood cells, so you will not need to have your blood tested if you take hydroxychloroquine. You will need periodic eye exams (every 6 to 12 months), because hydroxycholorquine can damage your retina (the back of your eye), causing decreased night vision or loss of peripheral vision.

Don't some patients get injections of gold for rheumatoid arthritis?

As strange as it seems, people have been using gold to treat arthritis for more than 50 years. We still don't know exactly how it works, but it seems to interfere with the functioning of the immune system cells that cause joint damage and inflammation.

Some doctors prescribe injections of gold (Myochrysine, Solganal) for the treatment of rheumatoid arthritis. This requires a weekly injection of gold into the muscle for about 22 weeks, and then less frequent injections after that. You might feel some increased joint pain for one or two days after the injection, but only with the first couple of injections. You should begin to feel the benefits of the therapy within three to six months. You will need to have your blood tested for signs of decreasing cell counts. If you have gold therapy for longer than six months, you might have to have your blood tested with every other injection. Other side effects include increased sensitivity to sunlight; irritation or soreness of the tongue; metallic taste; skin rash or itching; soreness; swelling or bleeding of the gums; unusual bleeding or bruising; and white spots on the lips or in the mouth or throat. You should not take gold if you are taking another DMARD called penicillamine, or if you have lupus, skin disease, kidney disease, blood disease, or colitis.

Gold can also be taken orally (Ridaura), but it does not work as well as the injections and it takes about six months to have any effect.

Is sulfasalazine a good choice for early stage disease?

Sulfasalazine (Azulfidine), which blocks inflammation, is another good choice for mild to moderate disease. This drug may cause a few more side effects than hydroxychloroquine, is taken two to four times a day, and takes two to three months to work. Sulfasalazine may cause the number of blood cells to decrease, so you will have to have your blood tested periodically. Other side effects include stomach upset, achiness, diarrhea, dizziness, headache, light sensitivity, itching, loss of appetite, nausea or vomiting, and rash. Sulfasalazine can also damage your liver, and people with kidney or liver disease should not use this drug.

I've heard of people with more moderate disease taking the anticancer drug methotrexate. Does this work well in rheumatoid arthritis?

For patients with moderate to severe disease, that is, with significant pain, evidence of joint damage on X ray, methotrexate (Rheumatrex) is an excellent choice. Methotrexate is used as chemotherapy for cancer patients. It interferes with the way cells utilize nutrients, preventing them from dividing, so cancer cells stop growing. It also inhibits the activity of the immune system, reduces inflammation, and slows the growth of cells in the synovial membrane. Methotrexate starts taking effect in six to eight weeks and has a good history of working in patients with rheumatoid arthritis. More than half of patients taking methotrexate continue taking the drug for more than three years, which is a longer time than patients generally take any other DMARD. If you take methotrexate, you will have to be tested periodically for liver damage and decreased numbers of blood cells. Side effects that occur with methotrexate include cough, diarrhea, hair loss, loss of appetite, and unusual bleeding or bruising. You should not take this drug if you have an abnormal blood count, liver or lung disease, alcoholism, immune system deficiency, or an active infection. It is also very important not to take this drug while pregnant, because it can cause birth defects. If you are thinking about getting pregnant, stop taking the drug at least one menstrual cycle before. Men who are thinking about fathering a child should stop taking the drug three months before.

I have severe disease. Is D-penicillamine a good choice?

Patients with severe disease, who have significant pain, damage to the joints, and damage to some of the organs, often are started on D-penicillamine (Cuprimine, Depen). D-penicillamine affects the function of immune system cells that cause joint damage. This drug is effective, but it might take up to six months before you notice the effect, and it is inconvenient to take, requiring increasing doses up to three times a day. It also requires monitoring of blood cell counts and urine tests to check for kidney damage. Side effects include diarrhea, joint pain, lessening or loss of sense of taste, loss of appetite, fever, hives or itching, mouth sores, nausea or vomiting, skin rash, stomach pain, swollen glands, unusual bleeding or bruising, and weakness. It's important to take this medicine consistently and not forget any doses, as starting and stopping can make the side effects worse. You should not take penicillamine if you have an allergy to penicillin, blood disease, or kidney disease.

Isn't azathioprine an immunosuppressive drug used to treat severe arthritis?

Yes, azathioprine (Imuran) is another drug used to treat severe rheumatoid arthritis. Azathioprine is an immunosuppressive drug—it acts by suppressing the function of the immune system, so that your immune system cells do not attack your joints. This medicine is taken one to three times a day and you should notice effects within two to three months. Side effects of azathioprine include cough, fever and chills, loss of appetite, nausea or vomiting, skin rash, unusual bleeding or bruising, and unusual tiredness or weakness. Azathioprine might reduce your ability to fight infection, so if you develop chills, fever, or a cough, call your doctor immediately. You should not take azathioprine if you have kidney or liver disease or are taking the drug allopurinol.

I've also heard that the drug cyclophosphamide is used.

Low-dose cyclophosphamide (Cytoxan), another immunosuppressive drug, can also be used to treat severe rheumatoid arthritis. It is used to treat people with rheumatoid arthritis who have severe disease of other organs or people with diseases like lupus. Cyclophosphamide is carcinogenic and very toxic, however, and requires careful monitoring. Side effects include blood in the urine or burning on urination, confusion or agitation, cough, dizziness, fever and chills, infertility in men and women, loss of appetite, missed menstrual periods, nausea or vomiting, unusual bleeding or bruising, and unusual tiredness or weakness. This drug might reduce your ability to fight infection, so if you develop chills, fever, or a cough, or if you have burning on urination, call your doctor immediately. You should not take cyclophosphamide if you have kidney or liver disease.

Minocycline is an antibiotic, but I've heard people are taking it for rheumatoid arthritis.

Minocycline (Minocin, Dynacin) is an antibiotic that has shown some benefit to patients with rheumatoid arthritis. It has not been approved by the FDA for use in this disease, but is available because it is used to treat infections. Use of a medicine to treat a disease for which it has not received FDA approval is called an off-label use. This means that your doctor can prescribe the medicine (in this case, minocycline) for you to use, but the manufacturer of the medicine cannot advertise that the medicine is effective in treating the disease (in this case, rheumatoid arthritis). Minocycline decreases inflammation, and seems to work best at the early stages of the disease. Do not take minocycline if you are allergic to tetracycline or if you are pregnant. It may also interfere with the effectiveness of some birth control medications, so be sure to tell your doctor about all the medications you are taking, even those that do not seem relevant to arthritis. A common side effect of minocycline is bruising.

A new drug, leflunomide, was recently approved. Is this a good choice?

Leflunomide (Arava) is a relatively new DMARD used to treat rheumatoid arthritis. It is a good choice for patients with serious disease, and it's exciting that new drugs are being developed, but it must be used carefully. Leflunomide works by affecting the immune system. If you take leflunomide, you'll have to have frequent blood tests and liver function tests. Side effects include skin rash, diarrhea, liver effects, and temporary hair loss. Do not take this drug if you have an active infection or if

you are pregnant or nursing. After you stop taking leflunomide, you have to wait for it to get out of your system,
or take another drug that helps clear leflunomide from
your system, before you get pregnant. Leflunomide can
even cause birth defects if a man is taking it when he
fathers a child. Arava is taken as a pill and costs about
$3,000 per year.

I've heard of a new class of drugs called biologic modifiers. Are they any good?

Another approach to treating rheumatoid arthritis is to
interfere with the molecules that cause the inflammation,
called cytokines. Two cytokines that are involved in
rheumatoid arthritis are tumor necrosis factor-α(TNF-α)
and interleukin 1 (IL 1).

Etanercept (Enbrel, manufactured by Immunex)
blocks the TNF-α receptor on cells—it acts like a
sponge to soak up TNF so that it does not bind to the
cells—preventing further damage to the tissues. This is
the first in an entirely new class of drugs, and was approved by the FDA in November 1998.

Cells have receptors for many molecules on their surface—you could think of a cell as a sphere with many
little docking stations on it, where different molecules
can hook up. Once a molecule hooks up at its receptor,
it can have any number of different effects on the cells.
When TNF-α binds to its receptor on certain cell types,
it sets into motion the actions that lead to inflammation.

Enbrel is actually a form of the TNF receptor. When
a person receives a subcutaneous injection of Enbrel,
some of this drug gets into the bloodstream. The TNF-
α that is floating around in the blood looking for a receptor is just as likely to bind to Enbrel as it is to the
receptor on cells. The difference is, if it binds to Enbrel,

it does not cause inflammation. So Enbrel decreases the amount of TNF-α that is available to bind to cells and cause inflammation.

The results with Enbrel have been dramatic. In one study, people with juvenile arthritis who were wheelchair bound and had severe side effects from their previous treatments were up, walking around, going to school, and participating in extracurricular activities. Overall, 80% of the people who took Enbrel experienced at least a 30% improvement in their symptoms. Even more striking, 40% of those taking Enbrel experienced at least a 70% improvement in their symptoms!

Enbrel is intended for use by people with moderate to severe disease who have not had a good response with other DMARDs. Enbrel can be used in combination with methotrexate. Enbrel is given twice weekly as a subcutaneous injection (an injection under the skin) and costs about $10,400 per year. The side effects of Enbrel have been mild, the most common being irritation at the site of injection. Enbrel can be given in combination with other DMARDs. People who have a serious infection should not take Enbrel, and if you develop an infection while taking Enbrel, you should notify your doctor immediately.

Can I take a DMARD if I get pregnant?

It is strongly recommended that women not get pregnant while taking DMARDs because these drugs may be harmful to the developing fetus. Methotrexate and leflunomide especially have been proven to cause birth defects, if either a man or woman is taking either drug when conception occurs. Use a reliable form of birth control while taking DMARDs. If you do become pregnant while taking a DMARD, tell your doctor immediately so he can decide how to adjust your medication or discuss other options with you.

My doctor has suggested that I take a combination of DMARDs. After learning about the side effects, combining these drugs sounds dangerous.

DMARDs can be used sequentially (that is, one after another) or in combinations with each other all at the same time. A combination that is commonly used is methotrexate, hydroxychloroquinone, and/or sulfasalazine. When used in combination, the dose of each drug can be reduced, which actually reduces the severity of the side effects. Combination therapy can be tricky, however, and should be done only under the supervision of a specialist. If you are not already seeing a specialist, and your primary-care physician is thinking of prescribing a combination of DMARDs, ask to see a rheumatologist as well.

In a recently completed clinical trial, called the COBRA trial, another combination of DMARDs was tested. In this trial, 155 people with early rheumatoid arthritis were treated with either sulfasalazine or with a combination of sulfasalazine 2 grams/day, methotrexate 7.5 mg/week, and prednisolone; the dose of prednisolone was initially 60 mg/day and was then tapered to 7.5 mg/ day by the sixth week of the study. Prednisolone was then tapered further and discontinued by 28 weeks, and methotrexate was tapered and discontinued by 40 weeks. The majority of those on this combination schedule felt an improvement within a couple of weeks after starting the combination therapy, and fewer stopped taking the drugs because of side effects than did those taking just sulfasalazine. After 56 weeks of treatment, the people on combination therapy had noticeably less progression of disease (joint damage) than did those on sulfasalazine alone.

These results confirm that combination therapy with DMARDs can be safe and effective in slowing the progression of rheumatoid arthritis. DMARDs are potent drugs, however, and should be used very carefully. Always talk with your doctor about side effects you experience, and do not change your dosage on your own.

How long before I feel the effects of a DMARD?

The DMARDs work slowly, and you may not feel the effects for weeks or even months, so do not be disappointed at first. Your doctor may prescribe a corticosteroid for you to take for the first couple of weeks. Corticosteroids act more quickly than DMARDs, but have serious side effects if they are taken for a long time, so they are a good choice to take while you are waiting for the DMARD to take effect.

Will I be able to stop taking all these medicines once the symptoms have improved?

You might be able to cut down on your medicines, but you will probably be taking some form of medication for the rest of your life. Most patients with active rheumatoid arthritis take an NSAID and at least one DMARD. Some also take corticosteroids. Once the disease is in remission (the symptoms have improved or gone away), your doctor may suggest that you stop taking NSAIDs or corticosteroids. Your doctor may decrease the dosage of DMARD after the symptoms improve, but it is important to continue taking your medication, since they control the symptoms of rheumatoid arthritis but cannot cure the disease. If you stop taking the DMARD altogether, the disease may flare up again and it may be more difficult to get it back under control.

How are COX-2 inhibitors different from current medications for rheumatoid arthritis?

As discussed in the beginning of this chapter, the COX-2 inhibitors work in a way similar to aspirin and the other NSAIDs, but are more specific for the enzyme that causes the inflammation. COX-2 inhibitors have an effect similar to that of aspirin and the other NSAIDs, therefore, but you have a much lower chance of getting an ulcer or kidney problems with a COX-2 inhibitor.

Should I change from my current medication to a COX-2 inhibitor?

You should speak with your doctor about changing from an NSAID to a COX-2 inhibitor. There are no dangers that we are aware of in switching, and, in fact, the COX-2 inhibitors are safer to take than NSAIDs.

Do not stop taking your DMARD, however, once you start taking a COX-2 inhibitor. DMARDs prevent the damage to your joints from getting worse, while NSAIDs relieve the pain and swelling. Like NSAIDs, COX-2 inhibitors will relieve the pain and swelling associated with rheumatoid arthritis, but will not slow the progression of the disease (see also page 45).

Can surgery help repair my damaged joints?

If you have severe rheumatoid arthritis and therapy with medication does not seem to be working, your doctor might suggest surgery. Your options range from minor repair procedures to complete reconstruction of the joint. In most cases, surgery will improve your ability to move your joints and decrease the pain. In most cases, it will also reduce the deformity.

Some of the types of surgery performed on arthritic joints can be done under local anesthesia, which makes the procedure much less scary. For example, synovectomy is the removal of the synovial membrane. This membrane can become thickened with long-standing inflammation, filling the entire joint space and leaving no room for the lubricating synovial fluid. Synovectomy reduces the pain and swelling and may prevent or slow down damage to the joint. The doctor can remove the synovial membrane using a procedure called arthroscopy.

Arthroscopy is also sometimes performed just to look inside the joint to get an idea of how extensive the damage is. With arthroscopy, the doctor injects a local anesthetic, and then makes a small incision in the skin over the joint. A tiny, fiber-optic viewing instrument can be inserted right into the joint so the doctor can take a look around. The doctor then inserts other surgical instruments into the joint to carry out the actual tissue removal. Once the procedure is completed, the tiny incisions are covered with an adhesive bandage (no long scars) and you should be able to leave the hospital within a few hours. Most people who have had this surgery can walk within 24 hours and are back at their normal activities within a matter of weeks.

Arthroplasty is a more involved procedure than arthroscopy and requires general anesthesia and a hospital stay. This procedure involves opening the joint, scraping off the heads of the bones that meet in the joint, and capping each with a metal or plastic head. The two caps are then joined by a spacer that acts as a hinge.

Osteotomy corrects bone deformities by cutting and repositioning the deformed bone. Resection refers to the removal of tissue—in the case of joint surgery it is removal of part or all of the bone in the affected joint. Resection is often performed on feet, wrists, or elbows, to reduce pain and improve function.

Sometimes it is necessary to actually fuse bones together, a procedure called arthrodesis. This is most often done in ankles, wrists, thumbs, and the big toe to relieve pain and allow the joint to bear weight again.

In some cases, the joint may have to be completely replaced. Artificial joints are available for the hips, wrists, elbows, shoulders, knees, and fingers. Joint replacement can have fantastic results for people who are nearly unable to move because of the pain and stiffness. After the procedure, which is major surgery performed under general anesthesia, most people feel much less pain and can get around much better than before. If you have a hip replacement, you will be able to put some weight on the joint after about five days, and after 12 days you should be able to walk using a cane. The joint will be almost normal after six weeks.

Joint replacement is not a perfect solution, however, as there are some problems with artificial joints. The joints may loosen over time, and provide a site for future infections. Development of better materials for artificial joints and better bone cements to hold them in place is a hot area of research, and many new options are becoming available (see Chapter 7, ''The Future of Rheumatoid Arthritis Treatment'').

It's getting more and more difficult for me to do normal daily activities. Are there ways to make life easier?

Yes, there are a lot of things that you can do to make the activities of daily living easier. It is also important to learn how to do things so that you protect your joints from further damage (see Chapter 8, "Living with Rheumatoid Arthritis," for more detail).

Can alternative therapies, such as massage or acupuncture, help with rheumatoid arthritis?

Yes, many people with rheumatoid arthritis find that massage, acupuncture, hydrotherapy (exercise in a heated pool), and relaxation techniques such as yoga are very helpful. Physical therapy can also help keep your joints moving freely, and some patients find that treatments by a chiropractor or osteopath can improve joint function. (See Chapter 8, "Living with Rheumatoid Arthritis," for more detail.)

I've heard of some people taking something called chondroitin sulfate and glucosamine for their arthritis. Is this safe?

There are some "natural" therapies being touted for the treatment of arthritis, and some people believe they work (see Chapter 8, "Living with Rheumatoid Arthritis"). Chondroitin sulfate and glucosamine are both natural substances found in the joint, and the theory is that if you eat them they will replace the substances lost in the rheumatoid joint. It would be nice if this approach works, but no one knows if it does.

These drugs—and yes, they are drugs—have not been

approved by the FDA, and have not passed the extensive safety testing that FDA-approved drugs undergo. I do not know of anyone who has been harmed by taking these substances, but you might be wasting your money. Talk to your doctor to see if he or she thinks it's a good idea for you to be taking one of these "natural" therapies.

Can diet help control rheumatoid arthritis?

Some people think that special diets can help relieve the symptoms of their arthritis, but scientific studies have not proven this theory. It is important, however, to eat a healthy, well-balanced diet, and not gain weight. See Chapter 8, "Living with Rheumatoid Arthritis," for more information on diets. If you are too heavy, your joints will be even more stressed. In addition, you will find it harder to perform the necessary exercises. It is also a good idea not to smoke cigarettes or drink alcohol. Alcohol can affect how some of the drugs that you might be taking work and also contributes to the irritation of the stomach produced by NSAIDs. In addition, your chances of falling or otherwise hurting yourself are increased if you are under the influence of alcohol.

A good diet includes plenty of fruits and vegetables and a balance of carbohydrates and protein. The omega-3 fatty acids found in cold-water fish, such as salmon, mackerel, and herring, might help alleviate the inflammation of arthritis, so try eating more fish and less red meat as your protein source. Do not eat too much fat. All people with rheumatoid arthritis, especially those on corticosteroids, should be taking calcium and vitamin D supplements to prevent bone loss.

FOUR

Are COX-2 Inhibitors Safe and Effective?

- COX-2 inhibitors have been tested in thousands of people with rheumatoid arthritis and osteoarthritis.

- The results of these clinical trials have shown that COX-2 inhibitors are as effective as traditional nonsteroidal anti-inflammatory drugs (NSAIDs) at relieving the pain and swelling associated with arthritis.

- The results of these trials have also shown that COX-2 inhibitors are much safer than other NSAIDs—COX-2 inhibitors caused far fewer stomach ulcers than did traditional NSAIDs.

- Because COX-2 inhibitors are very new to medical practices, the long-term effects are not known, but will continue to be studied even after the medicines are on the market.

COX-2 inhibitors have been extensively tested, first in animals and then in healthy volunteers, to make sure that they were safe. The drugs were then tested in people with rheumatoid arthritis or osteoarthritis to see if they work to relieve pain and swelling. The answer is a resounding yes—COX-2 inhibitors are safe and effective in treating arthritis!

∾ CASE STUDY

Edna is an 84-year-old woman who recently started having severe pain from her long-standing rheumatoid arthritis. This pain was preventing Edna from doing the things she normally did, including grocery shopping, housework, and light gardening. Edna had been taking piroxicam (Feldene) for the pain, but that didn't seem to be working anymore. Edna's 92-year-old husband has a limited ability to walk because he has chronic lung disease, so he is not able to help much with the daily chores.

Edna had been taking methotrexate for her arthritis, and it was working well for quite a while, but she recently started having trouble tolerating the drug. She had started to cough a lot and had severe shortness of breath, even when she wasn't exerting herself. A chest X ray showed that Edna had fluffy infiltrates in her lungs, which her doctor thought was most likely caused by the methotrexate. The doctor had Edna stop taking the methotrexate and promptly prescribed 60 mg of prednisone to correct the problems with Edna's lungs. Shortly afterward Edna began to improve—her breathing became easier, she coughed less, and when she coughed, she coughed up less phlegm.

As well as the methotrexate, Edna was taking several drugs for the pain, including Percodan, which consists of oxycodone (a codeine-like drug) and aspirin. When Edna stopped taking the methotrexate, the pain in her wrists and fingers became quite severe, so she began taking six or eight Percodan pills a day, which is far higher than the recommended dose. In addition, she was also taking two 20-mg piroxicam (Feldene) tablets a day, which is also higher than the recommended dose.

After two days of taking the high dosages of Percodan and piroxicam, Edna fainted while having a bowel movement. Edna's husband called 911 and an ambulance arrived shortly. The paramedics noted that the toilet bowl contained both blood and black stool. Edna was resuscitated by the paramedics and required transfusion of over six units of blood.

It turned out that Edna had severe bleeding in her stomach. She also developed serious problems with her kidneys—they stopped working—and she was sent to the intensive care unit at the hospital for kidney dialysis. After four dialysis treatments, Edna's kidneys started working again.

Edna suffered obvious bleeding from overuse of aspirin (in the Percodan) and the piroxicam. In addition, her kidney failure was most likely the result of a lack of blood flow to the kidneys either from the effects of the anti-inflammatories or the drop in blood pressure from her bleeding.

Edna's doctor has prescribed a new DMARD for her instead of the methotrexate, but she still has severe pain in her fingers and wrists. Edna cannot take aspirin or other NSAIDs such as piroxicam, ibuprofen, or naproxen for this pain, because she is at very high risk of dying from a bleeding ulcer or kidney failure. Her doctor is desperately waiting for the new COX-2 inhibitors to be available, because he thinks those drugs will relieve her pain without causing stomach or kidney problems.

Will many people have taken COX-2 inhibitors before these drugs become available?

The COX-2 inhibitors are currently being tested in thousands of people, and have been shown to be as effective as traditional nonsteroidal anti-inflammatory drugs (NSAIDs) in reducing the pain and swelling of rheumatoid arthritis. The COX-2 inhibitors produce far fewer side effects, particularly stomach pain and ulcers, than do the NSAIDs that inhibit COX-1. COX-2 inhibitors are also NSAIDs, but in this book the terms *COX-2 inhibitor* and *NSAID* will be used to distinguish between the two types of medication.

What NSAIDs were the COX-2 inhibitors tested against in patients with rheumatoid arthritis?

Celecoxib (Celebrex) has been tested against naproxen (Naprosyn) and diclofenac (Voltaren); and meloxicam was tested against piroxicam (Feldene), diclofenac, and naproxen. (Meloxicam is an NSAID that affects COX 2 more than COX 1, and so produces fewer side effects than the other NSAIDs. It is known as a preferential COX-2 inhibitor; see Chapter 2, "What Are COX-2 Inhibitors?" for more detail.) Celebrex and meloxicam are both effective NSAIDs that work against both COX 1 and COX 2 while causing fewer ulcers. Meloxicam is different because it is not selective, whereas Celebrex is selective for the COX-2 enzyme.

In one study, 1,003 people with active rheumatoid arthritis received a placebo (a sugar pill); Celebrex 100 mg, 200 mg, or 400 mg twice daily; or naproxen 500 mg twice daily for 12 weeks. All of those who received Celebrex at any dose or naproxen experienced significant pain relief at 2, 6, and 12 weeks, and no differences were noted among the doses. Joint swelling was also reduced in those people taking any dose of Celebrex or naproxen. In this study, one quarter (26%) of those taking naproxen developed ulcers, while people taking any dose of Celebrex had no more ulcers than did those taking placebo (4% to 6%).

Another study compared how well Celebrex stacked up against another NSAID, diclofenac, in terms of pain relief and ulcers. Both drugs were equivalent in their ability to relieve the pain and swelling of rheumatoid arthritis, but 15% of the people receiving diclofenac developed ulcers, as compared with only 4% of those receiving Celebrex.

In another study testing whether Celebrex causes as many ulcers as naproxen, 128 people took a placebo, Celebrex 100 mg or 200 mg twice a day, or naproxen 500 mg twice a day for seven days. The early results indicate that Celebrex causes no more ulcers than a placebo: No people taking the placebo or Celebrex had ulcers, while 6 out of 32 people taking naproxen had a total of nine ulcers.

About 2,500 people with rheumatoid arthritis have been tested in clinical trials of meloxicam. As with Celebrex, meloxicam was found to be as effective as piroxicam and naproxen, while causing fewer stomach-related side effects.

Have COX-2 inhibitors been tested in other types of arthritis?

Yes, Celebrex, Vioxx, and meloxicam have all been tested in people with osteoarthritis, with results similar to those in people with rheumatoid arthritis—pain relief as effective as NSAIDs and fewer ulcers.

In one study, 1,004 people with osteoarthritis of the knee received a placebo; Celebrex 50 mg, 100 mg, or 200 mg twice daily; or naproxen 500 mg twice daily. Pain relief was tested after 2, 6, and 12 weeks of treatment. At each testing time, people receiving either of the two higher doses of Celebrex or naproxen had significant pain relief. Those receiving Celebrex developed no more ulcers than did those receiving placebo. In studies involving Vioxx, 3,900 people with osteoarthritis of the hip and knee had relieved pain and stiffness and improved functioning when given 12.5 or 25 mg of Vioxx. The effectiveness of Vioxx was comparable to that of 800 mg of ibuprofen given three times a day or 50 mg of diclofenac (Voltaren) given three times a day.

Meloxicam has been tested in four clinical trials of patients with osteoarthritis, comparing it with piroxicam and diclofenac. In two 6-week studies, meloxicam was as effective as piroxicam or diclofenac at relieving pain and produced fewer stomach-related side effects. Meloxicam was again as effective as either of the two NSAIDs in two more studies, this time for six months, and again produced fewer side effects.

What side effects might I experience with COX-2 inhibitors?

COX-2 inhibitors are NSAIDs, and they act exactly the same as other NSAIDs, that is, they prevent the formation of prostaglandins. (See Chapter 2, "What Are COX-2 Inhibitors?" for more information.) Some of these prostaglandins protect the stomach from developing ulcers and some are involved in inflammation. Because the COX-2 inhibitors selectively prevent the production of prostaglandins involved in inflammation rather than those that protect the stomach, these side effects will occur at a much lower rate. No drug is perfect, however, and the COX-2 inhibitors are not without side effects. You might experience stomach pain, bleeding, and ulcers with COX-2 inhibitors, but the chances are much less than with NSAIDs. Other stomach-related side effects include indigestion, nausea, and diarrhea, but again, these will occur much less frequently than with NSAIDs.

COX-2 inhibitors can also affect the functioning of the kidneys, particularly in those people who already have some degree of kidney impairment. This can cause you to retain fluid and lead to a bloated feeling, or can cause dehydration. It can also cause changes in the levels of some chemicals in your body. Your doctor will probably perform some periodic blood and urine tests to make sure your kidneys are working properly.

Other side effects can occur but are very rare, including confusion, depression, rash, headache, and damage to the liver.

Remember, these side effects, and worse ones, occur with NSAIDs and corticosteroids, and much more frequently. COX-2 inhibitors really seem to be as effective as NSAIDs, but with much less of a chance of causing side effects.

A major side effect of Celebrex, however, is allergy related to sulfur. People with any kind of sulfur allergy should never take this drug. Vioxx does not have this unfortunate side effect. Also those people allergic to aspirin must *never* take COX-2 inhibitors in any form.

**How often will I need blood tests to make
sure that the COX-2 inhibitor is not
giving me bad side effects?**

With any newly available medication it is wise to
have your doctor check your liver function and do blood
tests for anemia every two months. With the new COX-2
inhibitors, it would be a good idea to have some blood
drawn for these tests at the end of four weeks after you
start taking the drug and then every six to eight weeks
after that.

The major side effects of NSAIDs are described in
detail in Chapter 3, "Other Available Treatments for
Rheumatoid Arthritis," and you should not experience
these significant side effects with COX-2 inhibitors.
With either traditional NSAIDs or the COX-2 inhibitors,
however, problems with the liver, kidneys, lungs, or
bone marrow are possible, but very rare. You should call
your doctor if you lose your appetite, feel tired all the
time, develop a low-grade fever, or have an unexplained
sore throat. If you notice that you bruise more easily or
bleed a lot from small cuts, call your doctor and ask to
have your blood tested. Anybody taking COX-2 inhibitors or traditional NSAIDs should also check for black
stools, which might indicate bleeding in your stomach
or intestines. If you are currently taking iron pills, your
stool might be black also, but you should still have tests
to make sure that there is no blood in your stool, indi-
cating a gastrointestinal bleed.

**Are the long-term side effects of COX-2
inhibitors known?**

Because these drugs are relatively new, there is not a
lot of long-term experience with them. They have been
tested, and found to be safe and effective, in people for

up to six months. The companies developing these drugs are very interested in finding out about the long-term side effects, and will continue to study them even after the drugs are on the market, so by the time you have been taking them for two years, there will be data showing the safety and efficacy for longer than that.

Will I start at the full dosage, or will I start lower and work up to a full dosage?

In the clinical trials, the patients started at the full dosage without any adverse effects. You will probably start at the full dosage, in order to obtain the greatest possible benefit. If you have side effects, which is unlikely, your doctor can decrease the dosage until you find a dose at which you still have pain relief but have no side effects. Current dosage recommendations for Celebrex are 100 mg twice a day for osteoarthritis and 200 mg twice a day for rheumatoid arthritis. The dosage of Vioxx is 12.5 mg a day for osteoarthritis, which can be raised to 25 mg a day if more pain relief is needed.

Will COX-2 inhibitors replace my current medications?

COX-2 inhibitors will replace traditional NSAIDs, such as aspirin, ibuprofen, or naproxen, and possibly corticosteroids, that you might be taking, but will not replace DMARDs. Do not stop taking your DMARD once you switch from an NSAID to a COX-2 inhibitor. And do not suddenly stop taking corticosteroids. It's very important to taper off your dosage of a corticosteroid so that your adrenal glands, which stop making natural corticosteroids when you take supplements, have time to start making them again.

Are there medications I should not combine with COX-2 inhibitors?

So far we do not know of any drugs that you should not take with COX-2 inhibitors. But you should not take a traditional NSAID with a COX-2 inhibitor, in case the side effects add up. You will not need to take traditional NSAIDs anyway, and may not need corticosteroids, once you start taking a COX-2 inhibitor. You should definitely continue to take DMARDs. The COX-2 inhibitor Celebrex has been tested for drug interactions with the DMARD methotrexate and the blood thinner warfarin (Coumadin). No interactions were found with methotrexate. In regard to warfarin, the manufacturer of Celebrex has recently sent doctors a "caution" letter about the use of Celebrex with warfarin. Caution is needed, however, in the use of warfarin with Vioxx or Celebrex, since Vioxx and Celebrex can alter clotting tests. For the most part, however, both Celebrex and Vioxx are safe to take with blood thinners such as warfarin. The companies producing these drugs will continue to test for interactions with other commonly used drugs. As of now, no adverse interactions have been noticed.

My doctor says I have to take aspirin every day for my heart condition. Will this be safe if I'm also taking a COX-2 inhibitor?

Aspirin is widely used to reduce the risk for heart attack and stroke. You are probably only taking 80 mg/day of aspirin for your heart condition, which should be perfectly safe in combination with a COX-2 inhibitor. At these low doses, aspirin can prevent blood clotting, but has no effect on inflammation. Fortunately, the dose of aspirin needed to affect blood and heart functions is much lower than that needed for anti-inflammatory purposes and should not cause any increase in side effects when used in combination with a COX-2 inhibitor. Make sure, however, that your doctor is aware of all of the medications you are taking, so he can make a decision on what is safe for you.

I like a glass of wine with dinner. Will I be able to drink alcohol when I'm taking a COX-2 inhibitor?

Alcohol in moderation (two or fewer drinks a day, a couple of days a week, for men; less for women) should not have any bad effects while you're taking COX-2 inhibitors. It is not a good idea to drink a lot of alcohol anyway when you have rheumatoid arthritis, because it can interfere with your sleep patterns (see Chapter 8, "Living with Rheumatoid Arthritis"). In addition, if you have an ulcer from taking NSAIDS, alcohol can aggravate that. So, try not to drink too much, but a glass of wine with dinner should be all right. We should not forget that the use of alcohol with certain DMARDs like methotrexate is strictly prohibited because a major side effect can be cirrhosis.

I understand that some antidepressants cause serious side effects when taken with certain foods. Do COX-2 inhibitors have these same problems?

No. COX-2 inhibitors do not have any known interactions with foods, and you do not have to worry about what you eat. You should, however, be eating a healthy, well-balanced diet to maintain a good weight and keep your energy up (see Chapter 8, "Living with Rheumatoid Arthritis").

The antidepressants that have interactions with foods are called monoamine oxidase inhibitors (MAOIs or MAO inhibitors). People taking these antidepressants must stay away from certain foods, particularly aged cheeses and wines, because the combination of MAOIs and these foods can lead to hypertensive (high blood pressure) crisis.

Can I continue to take my heart medication?

Yes, you can take all of your heart medications such as beta blockers, calcium channel drugs, and blood thinners. When the COX-2 inhibitors were first being developed, there was some concern that people would not be able to take them with blood thinners such as warfarin, but this has proven not to be the case. COX-2 inhibitors do not affect the levels of warfarin in the blood, and do not interfere with the action of this drug.

The COX-2 inhibitors have been extensively tested before they will be marketed, for their safety when used alone and in combination with other drugs. All of this testing has shown that these drugs are safe and effective when used alone and in combination with other commonly used drugs.

Bear in mind, however, that more drug interactions may show up as the COX-2 inhibitors are used by larger numbers of people who are taking several other drugs for other medical problems. The FDA and the companies making the COX-2 inhibitors will keep a close eye on how people respond to these drugs, and patients will be notified if any dangerous interactions occur.

I'm a smoker. Are there any known interactions between COX-2 inhibitors and nicotine?

There are no known problems between COX-2 inhibitors and nicotine, but you should not smoke anyway! Smoking is very bad for your health, and people with arthritis, in particular, should not smoke, because smoking has serious effects on blood vessels and bone. Smokers are prone to developing osteoporosis for a variety of reasons, and most people with rheumatoid arthritis have osteoporosis, either because of the medications they are taking (long-term use of corticosteroids can cause osteoporosis; see Chapter 3, "Other Available Treatments for Rheumatoid Arthritis") or because of their gender and age. It is recommended that all people with arthritis stop smoking.

How long will I have to take COX-2 inhibitors?

You may have to take one pill a day for many years, probably for the rest of your life, to control the pain and swelling associated with this disease. You probably will only have to take one or two pills a day, however, and should not have any of the stomach-related side effects that you may have experienced with NSAIDs.

Can I take COX-2 inhibitors if I have heart disease? What about neurologic diseases, kidney disease, or liver disease?

There are no obvious reasons why you should not take COX-2 inhibitors if you have heart disease or neurologic disease. In regard to the heart, inhibition of certain prostaglandins theoretically can cause an increase of blood pressure, a change in the body's minerals, a difference in the way blood vessels respond, or some headache, but there is very little information regarding these potential effects in people at this time.

Kidney disease could pose problems for people taking any drug, not only COX-2 inhibitors. Your doctor should be consulted before you decide to take this medicine if you have kidney disease. Experiments in rodents revealed that there were some kidney problems during the inhibition of some of the kidney COX enzymes. No drug is innocuous when a major organ in the body is challenged, but there is no comparable human data to indicate that the kidneys would be affected like they are in rodents.

In the development of the traditional NSAIDs, it was found that the early NSAIDs used for arthritis had terrific anti-inflammatory activities but they also had a propensity for making the liver enzymes rise; but this has not been the case with the COX-2 inhibitors. But people with severe liver disease should never take COX inhibitors.

Extensive use of COX-2 inhibitors will undoubtedly reveal new interactions with body systems and diseases, and your doctor will keep you informed of these new developments.

What should I do if I forget to take my COX-2 inhibitor for a day or two?

Do not forget to take your COX-2 inhibitor, not because you will have any side effects, but because your pain will come back! Try to remember to take your medicines on schedule to prevent rebound pain. If you forget, take another COX-2 inhibitor pill as soon as possible, and get back on schedule.

If I decide to stop taking a COX-2 inhibitor, can I just stop cold, or should I taper?

It is not necessary to taper your dosage if you should choose to stop taking a COX-2 inhibitor, but your pain will return! Be sure to talk to your doctor before stopping or starting any medication. If you are stopping because of side effects, your doctor may want to reduce the dosage or change to a different medication rather than have you stop completely. If you are stopping because the pain has gone away, don't be fooled—your disease hasn't been cured, it's just the COX-2 inhibitor working! You may be able to reduce the dosage in that case, but be sure to discuss it with your doctor before you make any changes.

FIVE

How Can I Get COX-2 Inhibitors?

- Both the COX-2 inhibitors celecoxib (Celebrex) and rofecoxib (Vioxx) are available by prescription; they are the first of several COX-2 inhibitors that will be available.

- Your primary-care doctor can prescribe a COX-2 inhibitor for you.

- COX-2 inhibitors will be more expensive than traditional NSAIDs, and may not be covered by your health plan at first. You are entitled to safe pain relief, so petition your HMO if you are denied coverage.

In early 1999, Celebrex became the first COX-2 inhibitor to be available by prescription in the United States, followed shortly by Vioxx. Doctors are very excited about this new class of drugs—the results of clinical trials suggest that COX-2 inhibitors provide excellent relief for the pain and swelling associated with rheumatoid arthritis, osteoarthritis, and many other diseases, without the side effects associated with NSAIDs.

What kind of doctors treat rheumatoid arthritis?

Your primary-care doctor can treat rheumatoid arthritis, once it is diagnosed and you are on appropriate therapy. If you have active disease (new or old), that is, if your symptoms are getting worse, your doctor might refer you to a specialist, called a rheumatologist. You can get a list of rheumatologists in your area from your local Arthritis Foundation office, the telephone book, or your HMO or insurance provider.

Can I get COX-2 inhibitors from my primary-care doctor?

Yes, your primary-care doctor can prescribe COX-2 inhibitors. Anyone who can write prescriptions—a nurse practitioner, primary-care doctor, or specialist, among others—can prescribe a COX-2 inhibitor.

Will my pharmacist know about COX-2 inhibitors?

Yes. COX-2 inhibitors are very new on the market, but they have been long anticipated, and pharmacists should be aware that they are available.

Have COX-2 inhibitors been approved by the FDA?

The FDA approved the COX-2 inhibitor celecoxib (Celebrex), manufactured by Searle, a subdivision of Monsanto, in December 1998. The Cox-2 inhibitor rofecoxib (Vioxx, manufactured by Merck & Co.) is also available. Roche Laboratories, Johnson & Johnson, and Glaxo Wellcome PLC also have COX-2 inhibitors in development.

How will my doctor know which one to prescribe? Are they all the same?

Celebrex and Vioxx are now available and several COX-2 inhibitors are about to reach the market. They are all chemically different, but act in the same way—by inhibiting the enzyme cyclooxygenase 2. If you switch to a COX-2 inhibitor in 1999, your doctor may not have much choice, only one or two will be available. After that, several companies plan to have COX-2 inhibitors on the market. Your doctor will prescribe the one he thinks will work best for you. If you are not happy with the results, tell your doctor and he will switch the prescription.

If I'm not happy with the results and want to switch, will there be any problems?

There should be no problems switching between COX-2 inhibitors. These drugs do not stay around in your body for long—waiting one day before taking the new drug should suffice to prevent any crossover reactions.

Will my health plan cover COX-2 inhibitors?

Yes, most major health plans should cover COX-2 inhibitors. However, because the drugs are so new to or not yet on the market, not all insurers have had a chance to weigh the pros and cons of covering these drugs. Doctors believe that because the drugs will be so effective at relieving pain and swelling and have a good side effect profile, most major carriers will cover their cost.

How much will COX-2 inhibitors cost? Will my HMO make me stick with NSAIDs, which are pretty inexpensive?

COX-2 inhibitors will be relatively expensive, more expensive than traditional NSAIDs. All new drugs cost more, particularly the first drug of a certain type to reach the market, because it is expensive to develop and test new drugs. The COX-2 inhibitors might be very expensive at first, and then once more of them hit the market, pricing competition will set in and the prices will go down.

Because COX-2 inhibitors will be more expensive than older drugs, many HMOs will probably not approve a switch to a COX-2 inhibitor from your traditional NSAID until you have a reason for switching. For example, if you have bleeding in your stomach or intestines or your kidneys are not working 100 percent, your HMO might agree to pay for the more expensive COX-2 inhibitors. You have a right to take safe drugs, so speak with your HMO if you are denied coverage for the COX-2 inhibitors.

❦
SIX

Beyond Rheumatoid Arthritis: Other Uses for COX-2 Inhibitors

COX-2 inhibitors are being tested in people with

- Rheumatoid arthritis
- Osteoarthritis
- Ankylosing spondylitis
- Acute lumbago
- Acute sciatica

COX-2 inhibitors may also be used to treat people with (but are not always indicated for)

- Other arthritis-like diseases, such as lupus erythematosus (lupus) and Lyme disease
- Sports injuries (indicated)
- Menstrual pain (indicated)
- Preterm labor
- Dental pain

COX-2 inhibitors may help protect against the development of certain diseases, such as

- Alzheimer's disease
- Colon cancer
- Other types of cancer

∾ CASE STUDY

Clara, a 26-year-old secretary, has the arthritis-like autoimmune disease systemic lupus erythematosus. She had been taking the corticosteriod prednisone off and on for about seven years, whenever the disease flared up. These flaring-up episodes consisted of high fever and pain in her lungs (called pleuritis, caused by inflammation of the tissue lining the lung cavity). Clara also sometimes had fluid accumulating under her breastbone, called pericarditis, or inflammation around the heart. Once so much fluid accumulated around Clara's heart that she was taken to the emergency room in an ambulance. Doctors there performed an emergency procedure called pericardiocentesis. They placed a needle through Clara's chest wall and into the sack that surrounds her heart to drain the fluid.

After that episode, Clara's doctor told her to take an anti-inflammatory drug like Indocin (indomethacin) to prevent inflammation. The doctor also prescribed 30 mg per day of prednisone for Clara, because some of her blood values were not normal. Despite the changes in her blood values, Clara's urine tests remained normal, meaning that she did not have the much-dreaded kidney disease lupus.

The Indocin took care of the chest pain and inflammation, but Clara had a hard time with the drug: She began to have terrible headaches and complained of feelings of "unreality." Her legs swelled to four times their normal size, and she became quite irritable. After a few weeks, she started feeling like her stomach was upset most of the time, and she had severe pains in the middle of her abdomen. She complained to her doctor that she had a "sour stomach"—she had acid backwash into her throat.

The doctor told Clara that for her sour stomach she should take the antacid Tums or the histamine blocker Pepcid (famotidine), which she could buy in the drugstore, and to take as much as she felt she needed. He told her to stop taking the Indocin, and he doubled the dose of prednisone she was taking. Clara was happy to stop the Indocin, but she was concerned, and rightfully so, about taking a lot of prednisone for a long time. She knew about side effects, including osteoporosis, that might occur if she continued taking this drug.

But what was her choice? She needed a medicine that did not have the side effects of either indomethacin or prednisone but would keep the inflammation of her lungs and heart lining in check. When the COX-2 inhibitors are available, Clara's doctor will immediately prescribe one for her—this is the drug she's been waiting for! Although she will probably need the prednisone to keep her immune system controlled, she will have an anti-inflammatory agent that will not cause the unneeded side effects.

What other arthritis-like diseases are COX-2 inhibitors used to treat?

The COX-2 inhibitors celecoxib (Celebrex) and rofecoxib (Vioxx) have shown great results in clinical trials of rheumatoid arthritis and osteoarthritis; Celebrex became available in early 1999 to treat these two diseases, and Vioxx is now available. Even though Vioxx is not indicated for the treatment of rheumatoid arthritis, doctors will likely try it to treat that disease.

Meloxicam is a preferential COX-2 inhibitor, that is, an NSAID that inhibits COX 2 much more than COX 1, and so has a better side effect profile than other NSAIDs. Meloxicam has shown good results in rheumatoid arthritis and osteoarthritis. It has also been tested in people with ankylosing spondylitis (an arthritis-like disease that affects the spine, among other joints), and it is showing good results in treating this condition. Meloxicam may also be useful in other rheumatic diseases that require a short but rapidly acting course of treatment. In one study, meloxicam used for seven days was found to be superior to diclofenac for the treatment of acute lumbago (inflammation of the muscles in the lower back). In another study, meloxicam significantly reduced the pain associated with acute sciatica (inflammation of the sciatic nerve).

COX-2 inhibitors have not been tested in people with any of the other arthritis-related diseases, such as Lyme disease or lupus, but it is expected that doctors will prescribe COX-2 inhibitors for many conditions related to arthritis. The research data on how these drugs work indicate that they will work in any disease characterized by pain and inflammation.

Have COX-2 inhibitors been studied as treatment for other nonarthritis diseases?

Recent data have shown that aspirin and other traditional NSAIDs may protect against certain cancers and Alzheimer's disease, and the results of laboratory tests have shown that inhibition of COX 2 is a key factor in preventing these diseases—that may be why NSAIDs have a protective effect. If that is so, the COX-2 inhibitors should also help prevent people from getting Alzheimer's disease and colon cancer, and they are currently being tested in both diseases.

Aspirin is often used to prevent stroke or heart disease, but COX-2 inhibitors will probably not be used to treat or lower the risk of these diseases, because a different mechanism is involved in the action of COX-2 inhibitors.

My mother has been diagnosed with Alzheimer's disease. Will COX-2 inhibitors help her?

It is not clear yet whether COX-2 inhibitors will be helpful in people with Alzheimer's disease, but there are some indications that it might help prevent getting the disease. Alzheimer's can be a very scary disease, not only for the person who has the disease but also for the family members and friends who watch their loved one change into a confused stranger.

Alzheimer's is a brain disorder characterized by gradual mental deterioration. It affects both men and women, beginning in the 40s and 50s. A form that rapidly becomes severe can start at ages 36 to 40, and a slower, more gradual form affects people at around age 65 or 70.

People in the early stages of Alzheimer's have difficulty performing simple mental tasks, such as balancing the checkbook or doing the housework. As the disease progresses, people with Alzheimer's have difficulty performing simple tasks, such as choosing clothing to wear for the day. They begin to not recognize people they've known for years. In the most advanced stages, people with Alzheimer's may lose their memory completely. They may also lose the ability to talk or use any muscles, including bladder and bowel muscles, and require total care and supervision. People with advanced Alzheimer's may become very aggressive and hostile.

It appears that COX-2 inhibitors may protect people from getting Alzheimer's disease, and these drugs may also prevent people who already have the disease from getting worse. But they won't bring anyone back to the state she was in before Alzheimer's set in, although some studies suggest mild improvement. Be sure to talk to a doctor about the possibility of treating your mother with a COX-2 inhibitor, because if it does work, you'll want to start as soon as possible.

How should the family treat a relative with Alzheimer's disease?

Your doctor will provide the best treatment possible, including medications to treat the agitation and possibly slow the progression of the disease. In the early stages of the disease, it may help your relative if you repeat things often, and remind her of things she's forgotten, in a simple, kind way. As she becomes progressively more ill, she may become extremely hostile. Don't take this hostility personally. Try to get away as often as you need to, and don't feel guilty about finding someone else to care for your relative—you need to have some relief too. Join a support group for families of Alzheimer's patients.

What are some of the current drugs used in Alzheimer's disease and how do they work?

Treatment of Alzheimer's disease is aimed at reversing, reducing, or slowing the mental deterioration that is associated with this disease. Many drugs are currently being tested, but so far none has been proven to cure the disease. Some drugs are available that can help improve the mental abilities of a person with Alzheimer's, especially in the early and middle stages of the disease.

One such drug is tacrine (Cognex), which has been shown to slow the loss of mental abilities in about 30% of people with mild to moderate Alzheimer's disease. Cognex works by slowing down the natural breakdown of a chemical called acetylcholine in the brain. Acetylcholine is important in memory. Cognex does not prevent the destruction of brain cells, however, and does not prevent the progression of the disease. Cognex also causes liver problems and is not used as much as it once was.

Another drug is donepezil hydrochloride (Aricept), which is also used to treat mild to moderate Alzheimer's disease. Aricept works by increasing the amount of acetylcholine in the brain. Aricept causes some mild, short-lived side effects, such as nausea, diarrhea, and fatigue, but can be taken once a day at bedtime, which minimizes these effects. Like Cognex, Aricept does not prevent the progression of Alzheimer's disease.

There is some evidence that vitamin E may prevent brain cell damage by destroying toxic molecules called free radicals. You can get vitamin E without a prescription, but be sure to talk with your doctor before taking it, since it can cause side effects. And remember, its effectiveness in treating Alzheimer's has not been proven.

Selegiline is a drug used to treat Parkinson's disease and is currently being studied in people with Alzheimer's. Selegiline also has side effects, and its benefits in treating Alzheimer's so far have been small and brief.

For postmenopausal women, hormone-replacement therapy may have some benefits in lessening the symptoms of Alzheimer's disease. Researchers are studying the relationship between estrogen and this disease, as estrogen has been shown to improve mental abilities in people with Alzheimer's.

Researchers are continuing to work on better drugs that will treat the symptoms, and, we hope, stop the damage to brain cells that occurs with Alzheimer's disease.

How do COX-2 inhibitors work in protecting against Alzheimer's?

Researchers are not exactly sure how, but they have some good ideas. People with Alzheimer's disease have protein deposits in their brains, called amyloid plaques, which are associated with inflammation. It may be that COX-2 inhibitors protect nerve cells from the damage caused by this inflammation. Two preliminary studies have shown that meloxicam inhibits some of the cells involved in inflammation in the brain. Another possible way that COX-2 inhibitors may work is by lowering the production of certain chemicals called free radicals, which may cause some of the nerve cell damage in Alzheimer's. A third possible mechanism involves a pathway, called apoptosis, which cells follow when they die of natural causes because they are damaged or mutated.

COX 2 is involved in apoptosis; therefore, inhibiting COX 2 may prevent the cells from dying.

My sister has colon cancer and is currently undergoing chemotherapy. Will COX-2 inhibitors be useful for her?

COX-2 inhibitors will probably not be a miracle cure for colon cancer, but studies have shown that people who regularly take aspirin or NSAIDs have a much lower chance of dying from colon cancer than do other people. Since COX-2 inhibitors act in a way similar to these drugs, doctors are hopeful that these drugs will also be effective.

The early results look very promising, and it will be truly exciting indeed if COX-2 inhibitors work in treating colon cancer. This disease is deadly if not caught early—and it is often caught too late. The current drugs used to treat colon cancer, 5-fluoruracil (5-FU) and leucovorin (LV), work in only a small percentage of people who have colon cancer, and the drugs have some pretty severe side effects. If COX-2 inhibitors, which have very minimal side effects, work, it will be a great advance in the treatment of colon cancer. But remember, these drugs probably will not cure disease in people who already have advanced disease, though they may prevent it from occurring or recurring.

Is there scientific evidence for why COX-2 inhibitors would work in cancer patients?

Some researchers have found a high level of COX 2 in about 90% of colon cancer tumors they examined. These researchers also found that cells making a higher than normal level of COX 2 are less susceptible to apoptosis, a pathway leading to the death of cells that are mutated or damaged. The researchers looked at cells from colon cancer tumors and found that they had very high levels of COX 2 and were unable to undergo apoptosis, a process that would normally kill any abnormal cells. Treatment with COX-2 inhibitors might allow the cancer cells to undergo apoptosis and die.

Researchers believe that COX 2 might be involved in colon cancer by causing the cells to produce chemicals called free radicals, which can cause mutations. These mutations, in turn, increase the chances that the cells would undergo genetic changes that lead to cancer. Treatment with COX-2 inhibitors might reduce the production of free radicals, which would lead to fewer mutations and less chance of cancer developing.

COX 2 also promotes the production of factors that encourage new blood vessels to grow near and into a tumor, which gives the tumor the nourishment it needs to grow. COX-2 inhibitors could prevent as many blood vessels from growing, so that the tumors would not have as much nourishment and would die.

Have studies been done to test COX-2 inhibitors in colon cancer?

These drugs have not yet been tested in people with cancer, but several studies have been conducted in mice and rats. The results of studies in rats have shown that rats that received Celebrex and were then treated with a chemical carcinogen developed 90% fewer tumors than did control rats (rats that did not receive Celebrex). The tumors that developed in the other 10% of the animals were much less hardy than were tumors in control rats. In another study, mice that have been bred to spontaneously develop colon cancer were fed Celebrex in their diet. These mice had only one third of the tumors found in untreated mice after three months of treatment. Meloxicam is also being tested in mice with colon cancer tumors.

All in all, the results of COX-2 inhibitors in colon cancer are really promising, and have researchers and doctors working in this field excited that a new treatment for a deadly disease is on the horizon.

Are other drugs available that stop blood vessels from nourishing tumors?

Drugs that stop blood vessels from growing, called angiogenesis inhibitors, are being developed and are being tested in people, but none are available for general use yet.

Angiogenesis is the growth of new blood vessels. This happens normally as the embryo develops and in response to wounds, to help the wound heal. All tissues need a good blood supply to grow, and because tumors consist of rapidly dividing cells, they need a really good blood supply to provide nourishment. Preventing blood vessels from growing near a tumor is an excellent way to stop the tumor from growing. Many research groups are working to develop good, safe drugs based on this principle.

One angiogenesis inhibitor that you might have heard of is thalidomide, which was marketed in the 1950s as a sleep aid and treatment for morning sickness. Thalidomide was removed from the market after it became clear that it caused severe birth defects, mainly because it inhibited development of the arms and legs. Thalidomide is not currently being marketed as a treatment for cancer but is used to treat some symptoms of leprosy. Thalidomide is being evaluated by researchers at the National Cancer Institute (NCI) to see if it is safe and effective for use in cancer patients. Given the rocky history of this drug, it is particularly important not to take thalidomide during pregnancy.

At least fourteen other angiogenesis inhibitors are currently being tested in clinical trials. Several of these drugs are in Phase III clinical trials, which means they are being tested in a large number of people with cancer to see clearly if the drugs are effective. These drugs are being tested in people with a variety of cancers, including lung, pancreatic, breast, prostate, colorectal, and brain cancers. Other drugs are in Phase I clinical trials, which is purely to test the safety of the drug, or in Phase II trials, which give an early indication of whether or not the drug is effective. To learn more about clinical trials of angiogenesis inhibitors, contact the Cancer Information Service at (800) 4-CANCER.

Angiostatin and endostatin are two drugs currently being developed at the NCI as angiogenesis inhibitors. Unlike most of the drugs currently being developed as angiogenesis inhibitors, angiostatin and endostatin are proteins that occur naturally in the body. These two drugs are currently being tested in animals, but, if all goes well, they may be in human clinical trials sometime in 1999.

Researchers and doctors are very excited that angiogenesis inhibitors will provide effective treatments for a variety of cancers, but the results so far are all in animals, and no one knows if these drugs will work in humans.

Will COX-2 inhibitors work to treat other cancers as well?

They may! Researchers have also found high levels of COX 2 in some squamous cell tumors (a skin cancer) and some evidence that COX 2 plays a role in breast cancer and head and neck cancers. It may be that increased production of prostaglandin because of over-activity of COX 2 is a common mechanism that allows cells to grow in an uncontrolled manner, leading to cancer. Whether or not COX-2 inhibitors will work to prevent or treat cancers is unclear, but researchers are excited about the possibility.

Why is it so difficult to find a drug to treat cancer?

Cancer is not a single disease—it is a family of at least 100 different diseases, all of which have a similar origin and progression. Cancers result from abnormal, rapid growth of cells, which form tumors and invade healthy tissues. Many strategies to fight cancer have been aimed at controlling the rate at which the cells multiply or at killing cells that multiply rapidly, but cancer cells can quickly adapt to their environment and become resistant to drugs. New strategies, such as angiogenesis inhibitors, may get around this ability of the cancer cells to avoid being killed by drugs, because angiogenesis inhibitors do not target the cancer cells themselves—instead, they prevent blood vessels from growing to nourish the tumor.

Will COX-2 inhibitors work in treating menstrual pain or sports injuries?

Yes, researchers think they are a wonderful option for women with menstrual pain and for people with muscle pain due to sports injuries. In fact, COX-2 inhibitors may be used for any type of pain associated with inflammation. Vioxx has specific indications for treating menstrual pain and sports injuries. For sports injuries, a high dose of Vioxx (50 mg a day for 5 days) can be prescribed.

I've heard that COX-2 inhibitors may help prevent babies from being born prematurely.

Yes, some researchers are investigating a possible use for COX-2 inhibitors in preventing preterm labor. After the egg is fertilized and the fetus develops, when it is time for the baby to be born, COX 2 is important in producing the prostaglandins that help the uterus contract and expel the baby into the world. In some cases, COX 2 acts too early, and contractions begin before the baby is fully developed, resulting in what we call a premature infant, or a "preemie." Doctors have made great progress in caring for premature infants, but in many cases being born too early is dangerous for the baby, who may die or risk not developing normally, and it is expensive and emotionally difficult for the parents to keep the baby in the hospital until the child is able to survive without medical help. It would be great for everyone if the baby would stay safe inside the uterus until near term.

One way to do this would be to prevent the production of prostaglandins too early, by inhibiting COX 2. It's particularly tricky to study drugs that involve pregnant women, because many drugs have adverse effects on the fetus. Indomethacin has been studied for the prevention of preterm labor, but it can cause some problems with the fetus, such as premature closure of a vascular connection called the ductus arteriosus and kidney problems. Meloxicam, which should not have those side effects, is currently being studied to see if it will work and be safe in the prevention of preterm labor.

∾

SEVEN

The Future of Rheumatoid Arthritis Treatment

In addition to the COX-2 inhibitors (see Chapter 2, "What Are Cox-2 Inhibitors?"), other new medications for rheumatoid arthritis are now in early stages of use:

- Arthrotec, a combination of diclofenac and misoprostol
- Etanercept (Enbrel), a biological modifier
- Leflunomide (Arava), a T-cell inhibitor
- Minocycline (Minocin, Dynacin), an antibiotic
- Neoral, a new formulation of cyclosporine

Other drugs and techniques being developed or tested for rheumatoid arthritis are:

- Anakinra, a biological modifier
- AnergiX, an immune modulator

- An inhibitor of phospholipase A_2, an enzyme involved in inflammation

- Infliximab (Remicade), a biological modifier

- Nitro-NSAIDs

- Zileuton (Zyflo), a leukotriene inhibitor

- Stem cell transplantation

- Better materials for joint replacement

Researchers are working very hard to develop new treatments for rheumatoid arthritis. It was only recently recognized that if this disease is treated aggressively in the early stage, some of the long-term damage can be reduced. Doctors are now treating people with rheumatoid arthritis with combinations of drugs to relieve the pain and swelling and to prevent further damage from occurring. No drug that is currently available will cure the disease, however.

∽ CASE STUDY

Henry was only 10 years old when he began to get very high fevers about once a month. Whenever he got the fever, he also felt very weak, had a rash, and his heart would beat very rapidly. After the third time this happened in as many months, Henry's mother took him to a doctor. Henry was put in the hospital and was tested for everything from heart disease to meningitis. All of the tests were negative, and, although the doctor was still concerned, the doctor sent Henry home with strict instructions to call her if any of the symptoms returned.

Two months later, the fever returned with the weakness and, this time, with severe pain in Henry's joints, so bad that he had trouble walking and could not sleep. Henry could not even stand to put on gloves or socks, because his feet and hands hurt so much. Upon seeing Henry in her office, the doctor immediately referred Henry to a rheumatologist, a specialist in arthritis. The rheumatologist examined Henry thoroughly—she gave Henry a complete physical exam, took blood and urine samples, and listened carefully to how Henry and his mother described what Henry had experienced over the last six months. The doctor noticed that some of Henry's organs were enlarged.

The rheumatologist diagnosed Henry as having a form of juvenile rheumatoid arthritis (JRA) called systemic JRA. This disease affects the whole body, which is why some of Henry's organs were enlarged—a rare and very serious complication of JRA.

The doctor told Henry to take large doses of aspirin to control the pain and swelling, and this worked for a while, but Henry developed a form of hepatitis, or inflammation of the liver, from the aspirin, so he had to stop taking it. He then tried a variety of other anti-inflammatory drugs, such as naproxen (Naprosyn) and tolmetin sodium (Tolectin), in the low doses recommended for children. The pain and swelling were lessened, but not to the point where Henry was comfortable. The doctor then prescribed the corticosteroid prednisone in addition to the NSAIDs, and the pain reached tolerable levels.

Henry's pain was lessened, but he wasn't at all happy with the side effects of the drugs. He now has ulcers from the NSAIDs and needs to take another medicine to treat them. He also developed a buffalo hump on his back and moon face from the prednisone. Henry is now 18 years old and in desperate need of drugs that will alleviate his serious pain and swelling, and also control the disease, without making him look so strange and feel so ill.

Henry's doctor is now going to try prescribing a tumor necrosis factor-α (TNF-α) inhibitor called etanercept (Enbrel) for Henry. This drug interferes with one of the molecules that causes inflammation and seems to prevent further damage to the tissues. The drug is very new on the market and is expensive to use, but Henry's doctor feels that Henry needs some strong therapy to alleviate his symptoms without causing disfiguring side effects. Henry's doctor is also eagerly awaiting the arrival of the new COX-2 inhibitors, which she feels will be a great help in relieving Henry's joint pain without aggravating his ulcers.

Are any treatments besides COX-2 inhibitors being developed?

The treatment of arthritis is an extremely active field for researchers, and several new drugs to treat rheumatoid arthritis have recently been made available.

Is anyone working on traditional NSAIDs anymore?

The traditional nonsteroidal anti-inflammatory drugs (NSAIDs) such as aspirin, ibuprofen, or naproxen work well at alleviating the pain and swelling of rheumatoid arthritis, but they have side effects that limit their use. Many people are working on NSAIDs to reduce the side effects. For example, Arthrotec (manufactured by Searle), a combination of diclofenac (an NSAID) and misoprostol (a synthetic prostaglandin), is an NSAID that produces fewer stomach-related side effects. Several clinical trials testing Arthrotec in people with rheumatoid arthritis, osteoarthritis, or ankylosing spondylitis have shown that Arthrotec produces far fewer ulcers than does diclofenac alone. This drug has been approved by the FDA and is available by prescription. Arthrotec works as an NSAID just like diclofenac but has the added protection of the synthetic prostaglandin misoprostol. The misoprostol supplies extra "good" prostaglandins to protect the stomach lining and prevent stomach ulcers, allowing the diclofenac to work on the pain and swelling in the joints. This combination is expensive, however, and misoprostol can cause diarrhea and bloating early on, so it is not a perfect solution to the problem.

Another area of research is the development of drugs called nitro-NSAIDs. These drugs are NSAIDs that also release nitric oxide, a compound that, like COX 2, is produced in small amounts by some cells and in larger amounts during inflammation. Nitric oxide may act together with prostaglandins to help protect the stomach lining from ulcers. Researchers believe that NSAIDs that release nitric oxide right into the stomach may help prevent NSAID-induced ulcers and may help heal ulcers that have already formed (see also Chapter 3, "Other Available Treatments for Rheumatoid Arthritis").

Are other drugs that interfere in the prostaglandin pathway being developed?

Yes. Another step in the production of the mediators of pain is an enzyme called 5-lipogenase, which is responsible for making a class of chemicals called leukotrienes. Leukotrienes are molecules that contribute to inflammation. One leukotriene inhibitor called zileuton

(Zyflo, Abbot Laboratories) is currently used to treat asthma, which is inflammation of the lungs. In clinical trials of zileuton in people with asthma, zileuton caused only minor side effects, most commonly heartburn and headache. Zileuton may affect liver function, so people taking this drug should have blood drawn and tested periodically. Zileuton interacts with the bronchodilator theophylline (used by many people with asthma), the anticoagulant warfarin (used to reduce the risk of stroke and heart attack), and the beta blocker propranolol (used to treat irregular heartbeats and angina). If you are taking any of these medicines, you should not take zileuton. Let your doctor know about *all* the medicines you are currently taking before starting any new medicine.

Another type of drug, called a phospholipase A_2 (PLA_2) inhibitor, is also being tested in clinical trials. This drug interferes with PLA_2, one of the enzymes important in the pathway that leads to inflammation. In fact, PLA_2 is the enzyme on which corticosteroids act. This new PLA_2 inhibitor is not a corticosteroid, however, and studies in animals suggest that this drug will not have the same side effects that corticosteroids have.

Are any drugs being developed to fight off the autoimmune attack in rheumatoid arthritis?

Yes. Another exciting drug that is being tested in clinical trials is called AnergiX. This drug acts to stop the immune system from attacking the person's own tissues, which is what happens in autoimmune diseases.

All cells have certain proteins on their surface, called major histocompatibility complex (MHC) molecules. MHC molecules are a family of proteins that help distinguish the cells of one person from those of another and help the immune system cells of one person recognize other cells from that person. It is MHC molecules that are responsible for the reaction when an organ transplant is rejected, and it is MHC molecules that help the immune system recognize bacteria or cells infected with a virus. In the case of autoimmune diseases such as rheumatoid arthritis, for some reason the immune system does not recognize a person's own cells as "self," and the immune system attacks those cells. For people with rheumatoid arthritis, the immune system attacks the cells that line the joints.

AnergiX is an MHC molecule combined with a small portion of one of the proteins that is thought to be involved in the autoimmune attack on the cells lining the joints. By treating people with rheumatoid arthritis with this complex of MHC molecule and protein, researchers believe they will force the immune system to accept the protein that it wants to attack.

Early studies of AnergiX have been promising, and this drug is now being tested in a Phase I clinical trial of people with rheumatoid arthritis who are currently taking methotrexate. This trial is designed to test how well people can tolerate the drug—what and how severe the side effects are—and to get an early idea of its biological effects.

Is there a vaccine that protects against rheumatoid arthritis?

Nothing available is a true vaccine, but we have seen some exciting results in early clinical trials with a vaccinelike drug called AnervaX. AnervaX is a synthetic peptide designed to block the stimulation of the T cells (white blood cells) that are involved in the rheumatoid arthritis disease process, preventing disease progression.

In a Phase II trial designed to test the safety and biological response of AnervaX, 53 people with active rheumatoid arthritis received the drug. To be eligible for the study, these people all had painful, tender, and swollen joints, despite taking methotrexate with or without oral corticosteroids. At the end of the study, the people who received AnervaX experienced significant improvement in the pain and swelling in their joints. Further clinical trials are planned.

Have any new DMARDs been developed?

Neoral (manufactured by Novartis) is a new formulation of cyclosporine that was approved by the FDA in 1998 and is available by prescription. Cyclosporine is an immunosuppressant that is fairly effective in slowing the progression of rheumatoid arthritis but has significant side effects. The drug is used by physicians who are quite familiar with its use and are alerted to its side effects. Cyclosporine is also used in preventing transplant rejection, and has significantly improved the rate of transplant survival. The most significant side effect of cyclosporine is kidney damage. Other side effects include muscle tremors, gum problems, excessive hair growth, and hypertension (high blood pressure).

I understand that an antibiotic is useful in treating arthritis.

Minocycline (Minocin, Dynacin) is an antibiotic used to treat acne and a variety of other infections. Minocycline was recently shown to modify the disease process in people with rheumatoid arthritis, producing significant improvement in the pain, swelling, and tenderness of joints. This drug is not FDA-approved for rheumatoid arthritis, but it is being tested in people with this disease (see Chapter 3, "Other Available Treatments for Rheumatoid Arthritis").

I've heard of a new drug called Arava.

Leflunomide (Arava, manufactured by Hoechst Marion Roussel) was recently approved by the FDA for the treatment of rheumatoid arthritis and is available by prescription. This drug slows the erosion of the joints and relieves the pain and stiffness associated with the disease. Like other medicines, leflunomide has side effects and occasional blood tests are needed to ensure that the drug is safe.

What are the drugs called biologic agents?

Biologic agents are medications that are designed to treat diseases by modifying their biologic processes. In treating rhematoid arthritis with biologic agents the goal is to interfere with the molecules that cause the inflammation, called cytokines. Two cytokines that are involved in rheumatoid arthritis are tumor necrosis factor-α (TNF-α) and interleukin 1 (IL 1).

Etanercept (Enbrel, manufactured by Immunex) blocks the TNF-α receptor on cells, preventing further damage to the tissues. This is the first in an entirely new class of drugs, and was approved by the FDA in November 1998 (see Chapter 3, "Other Available Treatments for Rheumatoid Arthritis").

Are there drugs that block IL 1, another molecule involved in inflammation?

Anakinra, which blocks the IL-1 receptor and thus prevents further damage to the tissues, is another biologic agent under development. Anakinra has not yet been approved by the FDA and is not currently available, but as of December 1998, a one-year clinical trial was underway. This clinical trial was testing Anakinra in people with rheumatoid arthritis who were taking methotrexate at the time but still had arthritis pain. People in the trial received either Anakinra or a placebo in addition to their methotrexate.

Are there other biologic agents being developed?

A third biologic agent is called infliximab (Remicade), which is currently used to treat Crohn's disease, a chronic inflammation of the intestines. Remicade is a monoclonal antibody that binds to TNF-α itself, preventing it from binding to cells and promoting inflammation. The early results of clinical trials testing Remicade in people with rheumatoid arthritis indicate that it reduces the pain and inflammation. The most common side effects are upper respiratory tract infection, headache, nausea, sinusitis, rash, and cough, all of which were mild. This drug is still being tested in people with rheumatoid arthritis. Remicade is administered by slow infusion pump every four to eight weeks and costs between $6,500 and $41,000 per year.

There are also products designed to remove certain kinds of cells from the blood in order to slow down the disease process. Other agents that block receptors on cells, such as one called the CD40 ligand receptor blocker, are being studied. Antibodies against certain kinds of T lymphocytes (white blood cells), such as CD4, have been shown to be effective in rodent models of arthritis. These drugs are a long way from use in people, but are helping researchers to learn more about what happens in rheumatoid arthritis and what might be done to slow down or even stop the process.

When will these new drugs be available?

Arthrotec, Neoral, minocycline, Enbrel, and Arava are all currently available. Talk with your doctor about whether one of these drugs might help treat your symptoms. Other drugs will become available when and if their safety and efficacy have been demonstrated.

I've heard a lot about stem cell transplantation in the news. Is this approach being tried for rheumatoid arthritis?

Yes, and it is one of the most exciting developments in the management of rheumatoid arthritis and other autoimmune diseases. But this procedure is experimental—that means it has not been thoroughly tested, and it also means that your insurance will not cover the cost. This procedure has had good results in people with severe rheumatoid arthritis who have also developed blood disorders such as neoplasia or aplastic anemia. These people have received a transplant of stem cells, which are really young blood cells removed from the bone marrow, either from their own bone marrow or that of a closely matched person. Once transplanted, the stem cells mature into blood cells and correct the blood disorder that has developed. In most people, the arthritis has gone into remission after stem cell transplantation. In some cases, it returns again, but these results suggest a promising future for stem cell transplantation. This procedure is also being tested in people with related diseases, such as lupus.

Are there risks associated with stem cell transplantation?

The cells for transplantation are taken either from the person with rheumatoid arthritis himself or from a healthy person with similar blood characteristics. They are treated very carefully and are tested extensively to make sure the donor did not have any transmissible diseases. The procedure itself is relatively safe for the person receiving the cells, but it still carries a 1% risk of causing death. This is considered by many doctors and patients to be worth trying, particularly for people with severe disease. Remember, though, this procedure is still experimental and will not be covered by insurance.

My mother had a hip replacement about 20 years ago, and it looks as though I will probably have to have one also. Has the technology improved at all since the 1970s?

Most people who have had a joint replaced because of arthritis have been very happy with the results, but in some cases, especially with implants performed as long ago as the 1970s, the new joint has become loose or worn. This can cause pain or make it difficult for the joint to work correctly. In the last 20 years, however, the surgical techniques used to implant the new joint and the methods of fixing the replacement joint in the body have improved so much that now more than 90% of replacement joints never have to be revised.

Debris from wear and tear on the joint is still a problem in some cases, and the development of new materials for joint replacement that would be less likely to wear is a very exciting field of research. Researchers are optimistic that new materials will soon be in use that will make replacement joints stay in place and last longer—for a person's entire lifetime, we hope.

❧

EIGHT

Living with Rheumatoid Arthritis

- You might experience fatigue, anger, or depression as part of your disease.

- You can modify your daily activities to minimize these feelings.

- Stress can aggravate the symptoms of rheumatoid arthritis, and it is important to minimize stress in your life.

- It is important to get a good night's sleep; get regular exercise; and eat a healthy, balanced diet.

- Alternative therapies such as massage, acupuncture, or chiropractic treatments, may also help.

- Many unproven remedies are advertised, including special arthritis diets; these have no proven benefits and are generally not worth trying.

- You can still travel and participate in family activities.

You've got rheumatoid arthritis. Taking a traditional nonsteroidal anti-inflammatory drug (NSAID) or a

COX-2 inhibitor (a newer type of NSAID) and a disease-modifying antirheumatic drug (DMARD) are good steps in the right direction toward controlling your disease. They are not the only things you should be doing, however. Learning how best to carry your body, protect your joints, and minimize stresses in your life are also huge steps in making life easier with arthritis.

ᨠ CASE STUDY

Igor, a 45-year-old Russian pianist, moved to the United States when he was in his mid-twenties. Igor recently went to see his doctor, complaining that he was no longer able to play the piano with his customary vigor, and that he felt severe pain in his fingers when he tried to play at all. He was no longer able to maintain his concert schedule—he had had to cancel several engagements and was not sure what the future would hold. He was depressed at the thought that he would no longer be a musician.

Igor was sure that he could explain what was going wrong with his hands. He felt that the symptoms were caused by a mosaic of problems brought on by the many difficulties in his life. He and his wife were having personal problems, he had an erratic concert schedule that took him all over Europe, the concert houses were often drafty and cold; in total, he felt he was under enormous emotional and physical strain, and this surely was the root of his problem.

Igor's primary-care doctor performed a complete physical examination, listened to Igor's medical history, performed X rays on both hands, and took blood and urine for some laboratory tests. Even before getting the test results, the doctor suspected that Igor had rheumatoid arthritis, so he referred Igor to a rheumatologist.

The rheumatologist listened carefully to Igor's analysis of the situation, and then answered his questions and explained how rheumatoid arthritis develops. Yes, the physical stress of the concert schedule and the coldness of the concert halls may have played a small role in making the problem worse, but they did not cause the disease. The emotional stresses of the separation from his wife might also have exaggerated the symptoms of the disease, but again, the disease would have occurred whether or not Igor was happily married. Likewise, his depression about not being a concert musician was understandable and may have made his physical condition worse.

The rheumatologist prescribed a nonsteroidal anti-inflammatory agent (NSAID) for Igor and suggested that he return in two months for another checkup. The doctor suspected that Igor would soon need treatment with a disease-modifying antirheumatic drug (DMARD) to slow the progression of the disease but was hesitant to overwhelm Igor at the first visit. Igor was also referred to a physical therapist to learn some exercises to maintain the mobility of his finger joints and to develop an all-over exercise program to try to keep him feeling energetic. The doctor also suggested that Igor talk with a psychologist to try to relieve his depression about the disease and Igor's sadness over the breakup of his marriage.

I'm so tired all the time. My doctor says fatigue is part of the disease. What causes this?

Fatigue is a sense of tiredness that can range from feeling mildly tired at the end of the day to feeling completely exhausted and unable to do anything. The fatigue that accompanies rheumatoid arthritis can be over-whelming and debilitating and can make performing the ordinary tasks of daily life difficult. Fatigue may actually be the most incapacitating feature of rheumatoid arthritis. It can make it difficult for you to concentrate and leave you without enough energy to perform your normal daily tasks, never mind perform well at work or go on a fun family outing.

Fatigue can be caused by the inflammatory process that underlies the arthritis—in that way it is a part of the disease—and, like the inflammation, it can be controlled with proper medication. The fact that you are tired all the time might mean that your medication is not working as well as it should, and you should talk to your doctor about changing drugs or adjusting the dosage. You might also have anemia, a common consequence of arthritis, which could be making you feel tired. Your doctor can do some tests to see if you have anemia, which can then be treated. The emotional stress of having a chronic disease can make you feel tired—if you think this is the case, your doctor can refer you to a psychologist or social worker for counseling. Or you might just be tired because you are not getting a good night's sleep or exercising enough.

In any case, it's important to try to control fatigue, since it can make your joint pain worse, affect your moods, and make your whole life more unpleasant.

Are there some ways to control how tired I feel?

There are lots of ways to control fatigue, and the best way for you depends on the cause of your fatigue. Your doctor can help you figure out what is the best course of action for you to follow. If you are feeling tired because of the underlying disease, your medications may need to be adjusted. If you are feeling depressed or anxious, it might help to talk with a psychologist or social worker, who can help you cope with the fact that you have a chronic disease. Or you might need some tips on improving your sleep patterns. It's very important to eat a good, balanced diet and to get a reasonable amount of exercise. If you need help with planning an exercise routine, your doctor can refer you to a physical therapist.

Sometimes I feel so angry about how disabled I've become. My feelings of anger are spilling over so that I've started snapping at my family and coworkers. How can I control this anger?

It's perfectly understandable that you are having an emotional response to the major changes that rheumatoid arthritis has brought about in your life. Anger is a natural response to the changes that have occurred—you have probably had to stop doing a lot of things you used to enjoy. Even getting through the minimal daily activities is more difficult. No one around you really knows what you are going through—even though they try to be understanding, they are not going through it. Your doctor, despite his extensive training, cannot provide you with a cure and maybe not even a medication that controls the symptoms.

But you are right: It's important to control your anger. Some people have negative feelings about themselves as a result of having a chronic disease—"I deserve to be sick because I . . ."—and end up feeling guilty. Others turn their anger toward others—"I don't care if he's not happy with my work, I'm doing the best I can." Some people completely suppress their anger, which can have serious physical consequences, such as increased blood pressure, increased muscle tension and pain, and increased fatigue.

The first step in learning to manage your anger is to admit that you are angry. You've already done that—you know that you are angry because you are not able to do as much as you used to and it is affecting your relationships.

The next step is to set realistic goals for yourself. How much do you expect to accomplish, given your new state of abilities? You are probably not going to be able to perform as well at work as you used to. So sit down and think about how much you can now accomplish. You are probably not going to be able to go hiking in the mountains with the family. So think about what kind of vacation you *can* take with them.

Then, figure out how you are going to set your plan in place, and talk with your coworkers and family members about your plan. Can you rearrange your work schedule or your office setup so that you can do your work more efficiently? Are there tasks you could trade off with someone or new skills you could learn that would compensate for things you can no longer do? Talk with your employer and coworkers about the changes that would help you remain a productive employee—having an open and honest discussion before bad feelings set in will go far in maintaining good relationships. Mary, a 37-year-old sales agent, found that one of her coworkers (with their supervisor's permission) was happy to give up some of her computer tasks and take on more of the sales visits that Mary found too tiring. With some changes to her office environment—a new chair, footrest, and armrest—Mary could easily do more of the computer work.

At home, talk with your family. See if you can reorganize household responsibilities so that you are doing less of the strenuous work. Plan family activities that everyone will enjoy but that will not tax your energy. For example, Leon, a 48-year-old father of three teenagers, was no longer able to ski with his wife and children, but he still accompanied them on day trips to the slopes, where he could take short walks in the woods and then relax in front of the fire with a book. At lunch and at the end of the day he was able to share in the stories about the day on the slopes, and the whole family was together.

The final step is to redirect your energy by changing your negative thoughts. Instead of thinking "I can't do this anymore," think, "Now I can do things this way," and consider it a success that you are able to still do some of the things you love.

Sometimes I find myself so depressed about my condition I can hardly get out of bed.

Many people with rheumatoid arthritis feel depressed. You might be in constant pain, unable to perform many of the activities you enjoy. How can you get everything done that needs to be done and still have any energy for a social life? Depression is not just feeling sad—it's an overwhelming feeling of hopelessness. Some symptoms of depression include lack of energy, lack of enthusiasm, forgetfulness, loss of appetite or increased appetite, difficulty sleeping or oversleeping, and lack of interest in sex.

It is important to manage your depression, not only

because you should be enjoying life, but also because depression can lead to further pain, loss of sleep, increased muscle tension, and fatigue. This can set up a vicious cycle, increasing depression and causing the symptoms of arthritis to get worse.

If you think you are depressed, talk to your doctor about a referral to a clinical psychologist or social worker. These professionals can help you deal with the changes brought about by your disease. You may also need prescription medication to help you break the depression. You might want to get involved with a support group (contact your local chapter of the Arthritis Foundation for information on support groups in your area), where you will find people with similar problems. Or just try talking with your family and friends about how you are feeling.

Most of all, it is best not to suffer alone and in silence. It is important to keep busy, doing things you enjoy with people you enjoy. Feeling good about yourself—by exercising and making sure you look your best every day— can also improve your mood.

It's difficult for me to get everything done that needs to get done at home. How can I resolve this?

Make a list of all the things you do around the house and at work. Try to figure out if any of those things can be eliminated or done less frequently. Now look at your new list and see if you can get family members to do any of the remaining tasks. Chances are you'll end up with a lot fewer tasks than you used to do!

It's also important to schedule and organize your day so you aren't crossing your tracks—if you have errands to run, do them all at once, rather than going out in the car two or three times a day. Leave plenty of time to get things done so you do not feel rushed, and be sure to plan some rest breaks. Finally, do not get discouraged if you don't get everything done. Many tasks can wait until tomorrow.

It's difficult for me to ask for help, but sometimes I have to. How should I handle this?

It's very important that you know what your limitations are and you ask for help when you feel you're not up to some task. If you overextend yourself, you could end up in bed! Talk to your family, friends, or coworkers before you need help, to alert them to the possibility of needing help. Let them know about your concerns. Letting them know ahead of time will make it much easier for you to ask, and for them to offer, when the time comes.

Should I try to get more sleep?

More sleep may be the key, but more restful sleep is probably what you need. A good night's sleep is important to recharge your energy stores and to rest your tired joints. It might help to take a nap during the day.

If you find that you are having trouble getting to sleep at night, or if you are waking up during the night, there are some steps you can take:

- Getting enough exercise, but not too much, can help your body be tired enough to sleep. Don't exercise too late in the day, though, or you'll be too charged up to sleep.

- Don't eat or drink too close to bedtime, or you'll be too full to sleep well.

- Don't consume any caffeine or alcohol at bedtime—a glass of wine might relax you initially, but it will interfere with your sleep.

- Start to wind down and give yourself a chance to relax one hour before bedtime. A warm bath, soothing music, a darkened room—all these can help you relax.

Will exercise help my fatigue?

Absolutely. While you might feel physically tired from exercise at first, a good exercise program builds muscle strength, which can help you carry yourself around better without tiring. Exercise can also help with joint flexibility. You will just feel better all around if you are getting exercise. It is important not to overdo it, though, and you do not want to hurt your joints, so consult with your doctor or a physical therapist to help you design an exercise program.

My symptoms often feel worse when I'm under a lot of pressure. Is that common?

Many people complain that their symptoms are worse at times of stress. It is not known whether stress actually increases the inflammation in joints or if people are just more sensitive to pain when they are feeling stressed. Whichever is the case, if stress seems to aggravate your disease, it is important to try to minimize the stresses in your life and learn some techniques for relaxation.

What are some signs of stress?

If you are stressed, you might feel irritable or angry, tired, anxious, or nervous. Your muscles might be tense, your jaw clenched, your hands cold and sweaty. You might have trouble sleeping or have no appetite. You might just feel a general sense of physical discomfort such as dizziness, weakness, headache, or muscle pain.

What causes stress?

There are actual changes that go on in your body when you are under stress. Your body produces chemicals that cause your heart to beat faster, your breathing rate to increase, your blood pressure to increase, and your muscles to become tense. Sometimes stress is good—the flight-or-fight response is an example of stress chemicals that are necessary for survival. When the stress goes away, your body returns to normal.

What actually causes your body to make the chemicals? It's a reaction to things that worry, scare, or excite you. One way to help minimize the effect of stress is to pay attention to what in your life may be causing the stress. If it is a personal relationship or a problem at work, see if you can improve the relationship or resolve the problem. It might be a good idea to keep a journal, so you can recognize patterns of stress.

What are some ways to decrease the stresses in my life?

Keep a journal to get an idea of when and why you feel stressed. Identify causes that can be changed, and concentrate on them. For example, if you are always rushing to get ready in the morning, getting up earlier, having your clothes ready the night before, and having someone else prepare breakfast and lunch might solve this problem. You might have to live with some stressful situations if you cannot eliminate them, so try not to worry about them for the time being. If you can get rid of some stresses, the others will not take such a toll.

Relaxation exercises can do a lot to minimize the effects of stress—they take your mind off the stress and help your body to physically relax. Yoga is a wonderful way to relax and get some good, deep stretching exercise at the same time. Or you could try meditating. Sit in a chair or lie on the floor, close your eyes, concentrate on even breathing, and let thoughts flow through your mind without letting any one thought stay too long. If you can do this for 10 minutes twice a day, you may find yourself more relaxed the entire day.

A slightly more structured version of this relaxation exercise is called guided imagery. Again, sit in a quiet room in a chair or on the floor, concentrate on your breathing, and think about a pleasant, comfortable place you would like to be. Concentrate on the details—the sights, sounds, smells, and feeling of the place. Think about how much you like the place. Relax. Continue to breathe deeply and evenly as you concentrate.

Before my symptoms got too bad I used to exercise a lot. Should I continue to try to exercise?

By all means, you should be exercising. It is important, however, to make sure you are doing exercises the right way, not overdoing it, and not hurting your joints. For many years, people thought that people with rheumatoid arthritis should not exercise because they would hurt their joints. It is clear, however, that exercise keeps the muscles strong, which actually helps the joints and keeps them flexible. It also gives you an overall sense of fitness, which helps with your mood, your ability to perform the tasks of daily living, and your outlook on life.

How do I know what types of exercise are good and what might hurt my joints more?

Your doctor can give you some idea of what exercises would be good and bad for you, and he or she can also refer you to a physical therapist. A physical therapist can help you design a comprehensive program of exercises tailored specifically for your problems. An occupational therapist can show you how to perform ordinary tasks without endangering your joints.

It's important that you not overwork your joints or muscles. Don't exercise too long or too hard, especially at first. Of course, if you were athletic and active before the disease flared up, you will be able to do more than if you were relatively inactive. You also have to take into account which joints are affected.

What types of exercises are good for people with rheumatoid arthritis?

It is a good idea to have an exercise program that includes a variety of exercises. The three main types of exercises are range-of-motion (flexibility), strengthening, and endurance exercises. You should choose some of each type; ask your doctor or a physical therapist to help you design a program.

Range-of-motion exercises help keep your joints moving in all directions. These exercises include neck, hip, and wrist flexion rotation; neck, shoulder, and hip rotation; knee extension; and other exercises that involve moving the joints. Most daily activities do not put your joints through their complete range of motion, so it is important to do these exercises in addition to whatever other daily activities you have. It's important to try to gently move your joints in all directions every day, even if they are swollen or sore. But if your joints are swollen or sore, do not vigorously exercise. It is best to wait until you and your doctor feel you will be able to exercise before you overdo it.

Strengthening exercises help maintain and increase muscle strength. It's important to keep your muscles strong to support your joints. One type of strengthening exercise is called isometrics, which involves tightening the muscles without moving the joints. For example, you can tighten your thigh muscles (quadriceps) or buttocks muscles (gluteals) without using any joints. Isotonics is another type of strengthening exercise, in which you move your joints to strengthen the muscles. You might not be able to do isotonics if your joints are painful or swollen. Isotonics are kind of like range-of-motion exercises, but they are either done faster or with weights added on. Isotonics can be very effective, and less stressful, if done in the water. Talk with your doctor or a physical therapist before trying any strengthening exercises, because you can damage your joints if you do them the wrong way.

Endurance exercises strengthen the heart, improve your lung capacity, and give you stamina—these are also called aerobic exercises. Endurance exercises can help you not tire as easily, sleep better, keep your weight down, and just feel better all around. Walking is an endurance exercise that is excellent for people with arthritis. It stresses the joints less than running, is readily available, and costs no more than a good pair of walking shoes. Exercising in water, either swimming or doing a water exercise program, is also a very good idea. Warm water is best, so the muscles do not tense up. The water supports your body, taking the pressure off your joints. Many community centers have water aerobics classes.

Bicycling is another endurance exercise that is well suited for people with arthritis. Try not to go overboard—a nice, easy pace on a route that is not too hilly is a good way to start. An indoor bike is ideal in terms of exercise, because you can set the resistance at whatever level feels best. Working out on an indoor bike may not be as much fun as riding with a friend, however.

Is it better to exercise in the morning or the evening?

It depends on the individual person. Some people do better in the morning and some in the evening. Try a variety of times and see what works best for you. Early morning is probably not a good idea for endurance exercise, because morning stiffness might make you less efficient and more likely to hurt yourself. Give yourself enough time to get all your joints moving well before embarking on your endurance exercise. It might be good to do range-of-motion exercises in the morning, however, to get your joints moving through the entire day. Don't exercise right after eating or right before bed. The important thing is to get in a regular routine—it does not have to be the same time every day, but doing something every day. If you miss a day or two, just start up again as soon as you can.

Should I try to warm up my muscles before exercising? What about cooling down afterward?

It is very important to warm up before exercising. A good plan is to do some range-of-motion exercises and light muscle strengthening before starting on endurance exercises. Otherwise you run the risk of damaging joints or straining muscles. Another good idea is to literally warm up your muscles, with a hot bath or heating pad, before exercising. That way your muscles are relaxed and less likely to get damaged.

Cooling down for 5 to 10 minutes after you finish exercising is just as important as warming up. Start your cool-down by continuing the exercises at a slower pace. Then do some gentle stretching. A really good way to end your exercise routine is to lie on your back on the floor, close your eyes, and just relax for a minute or two.

I don't often have a lot of time to exercise, but I want to get as much out of it as I can and I find myself hurrying through.

Don't hurry through your exercise program! Hurrying or doing too much too fast can result in injury. Start with only a light routine, then notice the next day whether your joints or muscles are sore. If they are, you did too much and should do a lighter routine next time. Make sure you take the time to do your exercises at a reasonable pace; you shouldn't be gasping for breath. This might be particularly difficult if you were athletic before the disease set in—athletes are used to pushing themselves as hard as they can. You cannot do that with rheumatoid arthritis, or you will end up with sore, inflamed joints. It is also important that your muscles get enough oxygen while you're exercising, so be sure to breathe regularly.

Sometimes it's hard to get myself motivated to exercise. What are some tips to keep me going?

It can be very hard to psyche yourself up to exercise every day, especially when your joints are sore. But you will feel better and be much better off if you do. Keep in mind that exercise is really good for you, and you will feel the benefits within a couple of days. If you do not exercise, you will also feel how that hurts you in a couple of days. If you are really sore or do not have the time to exercise one day, just do a little bit, enough to keep the routine going, and don't let yourself get stressed about it. As soon as you can, the next day or the day after, get back on your regular program.

Here are some tips to help make it easier to keep exercising:

• Work out with a friend. Arrange to meet at the pool for a water aerobics class or at the park for a walk. If you can't actually exercise together, call on the telephone to talk about how you did that day. Peer support is a great motivator!

• Make your exercise routine a regular part of the day. If you can work out at the same time every day it makes it easier. For example, try doing your range-of-motion exercises just after breakfast, then get dressed for work. Do some strengthening or endurance exercises at 11:30 A.M., then have lunch. And do more range-of-motion or strengthening exercises while dinner is in the oven.

• Do a little bit of exercise even on the days when you cannot do your whole routine. That way your exercise time slot will stay reserved for exercising.

• Think about how good you will feel when you're done.

• Do not think you have to do more than or even as much as you did yesterday.

My wife and I used to have a great sex life, but since I got rheumatoid arthritis I'm nervous about making love. Are there ways to get over this?

It's perfectly normal to have fears—fears about pain, about not performing well, about damaging your joints—during lovemaking, but there is no reason why you cannot have a fulfilling sexual relationship despite your rheumatoid arthritis. There are a few things you can do to help yourself relax. Try planning your lovemaking for the time of day when you feel best. For example, if you need a little time to get going in the morning and are too tired at night, see if you can make some time in the afternoon or early evening. It might be exciting to try a different time of the day! Take your pain medication beforehand, so it has time to take effect. Make sure you do your exercises, particularly range-of-motion exercises, during the day to relax your joints. Try taking a warm bath or shower (with your wife!) to relax your muscles and joints before you make love.

My husband and I would like to have a family. Is this possible now that I know I have rheumatoid arthritis?

Yes! Your disease should not stop you from having a family. Rheumatoid arthritis occurs most often in people in their 20s and 30s, which includes a lot of women of child-bearing age. There is no evidence that rheumatoid arthritis will affect your ability to get pregnant or have a successful delivery. Likewise, the disease should not affect the developing fetus—your chances are as good as anyone's of having a normal, healthy baby.

Your disease might even get better during pregnancy, which is good, since you might have to stop taking disease-modifying antirheumatic drugs (DMARDs) while you're pregnant—some DMARDs cause birth defects. You might also have to stop taking your traditional NSAIDs or COX-2 inhibitors. Be sure to tell your doctor of your plans before you stop using birth control, so you can decide what's the best course of action for you to take.

Will I be able to care for the baby?

Taking care of a baby is challenging, emotionally and physically. You won't be getting a lot of sleep, maybe for the first couple of years of the baby's life. Until the child can walk, you will be lifting and carrying a baby that might weigh up to 30 pounds. And there are diaper changes, dressing, feeding, and a lot of activities that might stress your joints.

You and your husband should talk about how this is going to work for you. If you can afford help for the first couple of months, even years, life will be much easier. You might have family in the area, but a lot of the work is going to fall on you and your husband—and he might be going to work all day, leaving you alone with the infant. If you are planning to continue working after the baby is born, you can only expect more stress trying to balance work and the demands of caring for a baby.

You can take steps to make things easier. Disposable diapers or cloth diapers with Velcro covers are easier to use than cloth diapers with pins. Excellent baby carriers can strap the baby to your body, taking the stress off your hands (although you still have to get the baby in and out). An occupational therapist can help you plan to make the infant years easier. And then there are the toddler years—a healthy, active two-year-old is hard work for anyone! It's an important decision for anyone to have a child. Be sure you think this over carefully, and are honest about your abilities, before you take the plunge.

Will losing weight help me feel better?

Losing weight if you are overweight will almost always make you feel better. You will feel better about yourself and will find it easier to do your exercises. The important thing about losing weight if you have arthritis is that the less you weigh, the less pressure on your joints. So yes, try losing a few pounds and see how it feels! Cutting down on fats and sugar is a relatively easy way to lose some weight, and a low-fat, low-sugar diet is better for you anyway.

Is there a specific diet I should follow or foods I should avoid?

Some people have touted special diets, which they claim almost eliminate the symptoms of arthritis, but there is no evidence that this is so. Rheumatoid arthritis is a serious, autoimmune disease, in which the joints are progressively damaged. No special diet is going to cure this disease. Their supporters may claim these special diets can cure the disease, but there is absolutely no scientific basis for their claims.

Because the symptoms of this disease are so variable—you might feel lousy one day and great the next—it is difficult to determine if your symptoms are affected by something you ate, something you did, or your state of mind. Some people might feel better, therefore, in spite of their diet, but not because of it.

There is some evidence that gout, a form of arthritis, can be set off by certain foods (see Chapter 1, "What Is Rheumatoid Arthritis?"). If you have gout, you should be careful of what you eat. Otherwise, eat a well-balanced diet, get some good exercise, take the drugs your doctor prescribes, and you'll be doing the best you can.

What kind of diet should I be following?

What is clear is that you must eat a healthy, balanced diet consisting of a variety of foods. That means a lot of fruits, vegetables, and grains, and some dairy products, meats, and poultry. The omega-3 fatty acids, which are found in cold-water fish such as salmon, mackerel, and herring, seem to have a beneficial effect on the symptoms of arthritis. You might consider, therefore, having fish a couple of nights a week and cutting down on red meat.

Make sure you get enough calcium and vitamin D in your diet, to prevent too much bone loss and to ward off osteoporosis (thinning of the bones). People with osteoporosis are much more susceptible to broken bones. Calcium is one of the main building blocks of bones, and you should be getting 1,000 to 1,500 mg per day in your diet to keep your bones strong. Milk, cheese, green leafy vegetables, and cantaloupe are good sources of calcium. Vitamin D is important in keeping bones strong because it helps your body absorb calcium from your intestines—without vitamin D you could eat all the calcium you wanted, but most of it would go right back out again without ever seeing the bones. Liver, fish oil, and dairy products contain a lot of vitamin D. You should be getting 400 IU (international units) of this vitamin every day.

I've heard a lot about other herbal remedies. Do any of those really work?

There is no scientific evidence that any of the "unproven remedies" for arthritis really work. Some might even be dangerous. But even those that are not dangerous can cause people to waste their time and money and can create a harmful situation if their use delays the start of legitimate therapy. People with arthritis spend billions of dollars, and a lot of hope, on untested cures, and may not be seeking appropriate medical care.

Anything that you inject or take by mouth could have an effect not only on your illness but also on your general well-being. Some unproven remedies that could be harmful but probably will not have much of an effect beyond a placebo effect (feeling temporarily better after a treatment) include the following:

• Wearing a copper bracelet

• Drinking elderberry wine

• Applying the solvent DMSO (dimethyl sulfoxide) to your sore joints

• Spraying the lubricant WD-40 on your joints

• Injecting snake venom (which can be dangerous!)

• Taking megadoses of vitamins (although it is a good idea to take a daily multivitamin supplement)

Here are some ways to spot potentially risky treatments:

• Avoid remedies that offer a cure. If this were true, it would be widely publicized in the legitimate medical press and would probably be marketed by a major drug company. Generally these so-called "cures" are never exposed to peer review (review by other researchers) and scientific scrutiny. When you have doubts about a "cure," ask where the data were published and if the journal is widely accepted.

- Again, be leery if there is no scientific evidence (in reputable medical journals) that the product does what it says. If patient testimonials are the only evidence of the product's effectiveness, it hasn't been adequately proven.

- Be very nervous if the supplier provides only a P.O. box number in the advertisements. A reputable company will provide a formal address.

- Don't go for anything that is outrageously expensive! You don't always get what you pay for.

- Don't take anything that does not have a complete list of ingredients on the package. Many products contain contaminants that can be harmful.

- If it is a service that's being offered, don't trust anyone who wants cash and will not take insurance as payment.

- Don't trust staff at a program that claim that the medical community is conspiring to suppress their treatments.

- Don't bother going for treatments offered in a distant or exotic location.

- Nothing is going to offer an overnight cure. Do not believe anyone touting this claim. Remember when an arthritis cure is found, it will be big news and not something that will have to beg an audience.

Can alternative therapies, such as massage or acupuncture, help with rheumatoid arthritis?

Yes. Massage can help increase blood flow around the joint and loosen scar tissue that has formed, making the joints more able to move freely. Acupuncture may also relieve the pain of arthritis. No one really knows how acupuncture works, but some people think that sticking the long, thin needles into the body causes painkilling substances made in the brain to be released into the bloodstream.

Hydrotherapy, or exercise in a heated swimming pool, is also very good. Floating in the water takes some of the pressure off your joints and allows you to relax. Heat treatments, such as a heating pad or hot water bottle put right on the affected joint, improve the blood flow in the region of the joint, relieving the pain and swelling.

Physical therapy is another excellent way to help keep the joints moving freely. The physical therapist can help you design an exercise program to do at home also. Some people find that treatments by a chiropractor or osteopath also help restore normal function in the joints.

I used to love to cook, but now I'm so tired and lethargic I can hardly get up the energy for a bowl of cereal, never mind a healthy, balanced meal.

It can seem difficult to plan, shop for, and cook a healthy well-balanced meal, especially when you are tired and in pain. It is easier than you might think, however. Forget the old days, when you might have spent hours preparing a multicourse dinner with sauces on everything. Think simple and fresh. Have a supply of fresh fruit and vegetables around the house—then just pick one up and nibble on it at snack time! Steamed vegetables with olive oil or butter are easy to prepare. Broiled or grilled fish with bulgur or rice makes a delicious dinner. Buy prechopped vegetables and salads at the supermarket. Browse through cookbooks in the bookstore for ones that supply simple, quick meal plans. If you are still having trouble, ask your doctor to refer you to an occupational therapist, who can give you advice on making cooking easier.

Can I drink alcohol?

Cutting out, or at least down on, alcohol is strongly recommended. Alcohol can have adverse effects if combined with some medications. If you are taking an NSAID such as ibuprofen or aspirin, you are at risk for developing an ulcer, and alcohol can increase your chances. Alcohol combined with acetaminophen or methotrexate can cause liver damage. And alcohol can also aggravate gout. If you are trying to lose weight, cutting out alcohol can make you lose a few pounds quickly. Talk to your doctor about drinking alcohol, particularly with regards to how it affects your medication.

I'm really afraid I'm going to hurt my joints. Are there ways to protect them as I go about my daily routine?

It's a good idea to learn how to modify your activities so you don't put too much stress on your joints. Overusing your joints can make the pain much worse. Try to organize your activities so that you do a more physically demanding task, then one that requires you to sit, and then another physically demanding one. Interspersing activities this way allows your joints to work a little, then rest a little. Also, when sitting for a long period of time, change your position frequently and move your joints a little so they do not get stiff.

Three commonly used methods of joint protection are joint positioning, using assistive devices, and controlling your weight.

Joint positioning means using your joints more efficiently to reduce the amount of stress put on them—use the big muscles and strong joints to lift and carry. For example, use your forearms and the palms of your hands instead of your fingers when you carry things. Bend your knees when you want to pick something up off the floor, rather than bending at the waist, so that you are using your quadricep muscles (thighs) rather than your back.

Assistive devices range from simple devices such as utensils with large handles to canes, crutches, and walkers. A variety of devices are available that can make the simplest of tasks much easier and less stressful on your joints. These include lever faucets, lever door-handles, special pizza cutters and can openers, long-handled shoehorns and bath brushes, and electric toothbrushes and razors. Splints are also a useful aid for people with rheumatoid arthritis.

Control your weight and exercise to minimize stresses on your joints, as is discussed earlier in this chapter.

How do splints help someone with rheumatoid arthritis?

Splints are a useful aid for people with rheumatoid arthritis. These devices can keep the joint from moving, thus allowing the swelling to settle down. They can also hold the joint at the best angle to allow function of a joint. An example would be a hand-wrist splint that would allow you to work at the computer or even play the piano.

My doctor told me to improve my posture. Why is this important?

Practicing good posture means putting your body in the most efficient and least stressful position. This can keep you from getting tired and can take stress off of your affected joints.

When you stand, imagine a straight line connecting your ears, shoulders, hips, knees, and heels. Stand with your knees slightly bent, your stomach muscles tight, your buttocks tucked in, your shoulders held back and down (but not tense), and your chin tucked slightly. Stand with your feet slightly apart and one slightly ahead of the other to improve your balance. Now take a deep breath and relax. It may help to lean against a wall or put one foot on a stool if you have to stand for a long time.

When you're sitting, your spine should be stable and supported. You might want to place a rolled-up towel or a pillow behind your lower back; special low-back cushions are also available. Keep your hips, knees, and ankles at a 90-degree angle, hold your shoulders down and back (but not tense), and tuck your chin slightly. Keep your shoulders relaxed, your elbows at a 90-degree angle or lower, and your wrists straight. If you work at a desk, get an adjustable chair so you can position yourself carefully. You might need a stool for your feet.

When lying down on your back, keep a small towel rolled up in your pillowcase, or use a cervical pillow, to protect your neck. Don't use pillows under your knees. When lying on your side, use several pillows or a large body pillow to support your arms and legs.

What does it mean to "distribute your load" better?

Distributing your load is related to good posture. It means spreading your weight around to as many major muscle groups as possible, so you are not overstressing any one joint. For example, use a purse with a shoulder strap, or a backpack, rather than a hand-held bag. This protects your elbow, wrist, and finger joints, and also keeps your back and hips in better alignment. Use your arms instead of your hands, and the palms of your hands instead of your fingers, to lift or carry things. When climbing stairs, start with your stronger leg, and when going down, lead with your weaker leg.

Most daily activities are difficult for me, even getting dressed. What are some ways to make life easier?

There are many things you can do to make your life easier and protect your joints while performing the tasks of daily living. Here is a list of suggestions. For more information contact your local Arthritis Foundation and ask for their brochure *Self-Help Manual for Patients with Arthritis*, which is available for a nominal fee. For help designing a routine for your specific needs, ask your doctor to refer you to an occupational therapist.

- Wear loose-fitting clothes with larger neck and arm holes.

- Wear clothes with front openings and elastic waist.

- Wear clothes with large pockets so you can carry things around with you and don't have to retrace your steps.

- Use long-handled shoehorns and sock aids.

- Wear pretied neckties.

- Wear slip-on shoes or shoes with Velcro closures.

- Use buttoning aids or replace buttons with Velcro closures.

- Use zipper pulls or add a loop or chain to the zipper to make it easier to grasp.

- Sit down to get dressed.

How about some tips on cooking and cleaning up afterward?

There are many ways you can make things easier in the kitchen. Remember to leave plenty of time for cooking and cleaning up, or prepare meals ahead of time, so you are not under a lot of pressure at meal time.

- Plan meals ahead of time to lessen last-minute tasks.

- Use electric appliances, such as a food processor, blender, mixer, crockpot, can opener, microwave oven, and dishwasher to save time and minimize the stress on your joints.

- Use disposable aluminum baking pans or use the same pan for cooking and serving to make cleanup easier.

- Sprays pans with nonstick vegetable spray or line them with foil to make cleanup easier.

- Store large appliances and commonly used items on the counter.

- Store heavier items at waist level so you don't have to reach for them. Use a grabber to reach for lighter items stored above.

- Sit down while preparing food, either at the table or on a high stool at the counter.

- Use a wheeled cart to transport items.

- Place a mixing bowl down low—in the sink, for example—while stirring.

- Fasten large cloth loops to the refrigerator door and drawer handles. Stick your arm through and use your forearm, rather than your fingers, to pull.

- Purchase a good, sharp knife. The initial expense is well worth how much easier it will cut.

- Use a garbage can with a pedal.

Laundry and housekeeping are particularly difficult. Are there some ways to make these easier?

Someone has to do the laundry and housecleaning, but it probably does not have to be done as often as you think. Try to clean only the well-trafficked areas often, leaving the less noticeable cleaning for another day. Do only one major cleaning task each day—do not try to do the vacuuming and clean the bathroom in the same day. Or, enlist help from family members, giving away the strenuous tasks. Here are some additional tips:

- Use separate laundry baskets for light and dark clothes, so you don't have to sort before washing. After washing, fold clothes in separate baskets for each family member to put away.

- Use a rolling laundry cart.

- Sit to sort and fold clothes.

- Use a long-handled mop to clean floors, preferably a sponge mop with a squeezer.

- Use a long-handled duster.

- Dust with a mitt or an old sock, using the palm of your hand in a circular motion.

- Store separate cleaning supplies upstairs and downstairs. Keep supplies on a rolling cart to move from room to room.

- Keep supplies on easy-to-reach shelves.

- Use an automatic toilet bowl cleaner.

- Use spray-on mildew remover so you won't have to scrub.

- Let dishes air dry rather than drying with a towel.

I'm afraid I'm going to fall in the bathroom. Are there ways to make myself safer?

You are right, there are lots of opportunities to fall and get hurt in the bathroom. You can take several steps to make your bathroom much safer and more convenient to use.

- Use a raised toilet seat to make it easier to get up and down.

- Install hand rails next to the toilet and in the bathtub or shower stall.

- Use a rubber mat or grip strips in the tub or shower.

- Install a bench or seat in your tub or shower stall.

- Wash with a bath mitt or long-handled brush.

- Use an extra-long-handled brush or comb, and build up the handle with foam to make it easier to grip.

- Install lever handles on faucets.

- Use pump-style toothpaste, or squeeze the tube with your palm on the counter.

- Use an electric toothbrush.

- Place a free-standing mirror in a convenient location so you don't have to stand at the sink to shave or apply makeup.

- Keep towels within easy reach.

At work, some of the simplest tasks are difficult because of my joint pain. What are some tips on making things easier at the office?

The workplace can be particularly difficult because you do not want to seem helpless or unable to complete tasks in front of your boss or coworkers. Fortunately, you can rearrange your office and procedures in several ways to make things a lot easier.

- Use a chair that can be easily adjusted.

- Use a footrest.

- Keep all supplies in easy reach.

- Use a lateral filing cabinet to avoid having to reach.

- Keep your current work in a vertical file on your desk.

- Install wrist rests on your keyboard.

- Install a glareproof screen on your computer monitor

so you don't have to strain your neck to read the screen.

It's difficult for me to get around, even in the car. Are there things I can do to make driving easier?

It's nice to be able to get around, and the car can be a big help. Here are some suggestions for making driving easier.

- Use a car with power steering, power windows, and power seat controls.

- Other helpful features in many cars include tiltable steering wheels, cruise control, and adjustable head rests.

- Use a key holder to make turning the key easier, which can be hard on painful finger joints.

- Have lever-type door handles installed to make opening the doors easier.

- Install a wide-angle mirror to avoid straining your neck.

- When on long trips, stop frequently to get out and stretch.

- Pack snacks and beverages so you can take your medicines while on a long trip.

- In cold weather, have someone else warm up the car before you get in. Or you might be able to use an automatic car starter.

- Install grab bars on the roof to help you get in and out of the car.

I'm planning a vacation with my family, but I'm nervous about being away from my doctor for a long time.

There is no reason that you can't take a vacation—and enjoy yourself—despite your disease. Be sure you talk with your doctor about your vacation plans to make sure you are not going to overextend yourself. Your doctor can also give you the names and numbers of some doctors where you are going, just in case you need a doctor's care while you are away. See "Resources" (page 213) for information on trips especially designed for people who have trouble getting around.

Be sure to take along enough medication! It is a good idea to take one or two weeks' worth of extra medicine, just in case you run out, or your medicine gets lost or damaged. Ask your doctor for an extra prescription to bring along as well. If you're flying, carry your medication on the plane with you—do not pack it in your luggage. You don't want your medicine ending up in a different city! If you're driving, keep your medicine in the car, not in the trunk, where it might be exposed to temperature extremes.

Write down a description of your medical problems and a list of your medicines, and keep it in your purse, wallet, or pocket. If anything happens to you, you want immediate attention and you don't want to miss your medications. A Medic Alert bracelet can be helpful in this respect. For more information about acquiring a Medic Alert bracelet, see page 215.

I'm planning a trip to Europe for our anniversary, but I'm nervous about getting around. Are there things I can do to make the trip run more smoothly?

A long and involved trip can be difficult for someone with rheumatoid arthritis, but with good planning, this could be a great vacation (see "Resources," page 213, for brochures on traveling with a disability). Remember, don't try to overdo it! Visiting museum after museum can be very tiring, and you don't want to spend the latter half of your vacation in bed. Many hotels are especially equipped for people with special needs and requests. Ask your travel agent to recommend good hotels and check to make sure there is an elevator and grab bars in the bathroom. If you need a wheelchair, ask if the room and bathroom are wheelchair-accessible. Plan to intersperse more strenuous activities, such as hikes or museum visits, with more leisurely ones, such as an afternoon in a park or a nice luncheon.

Call the airline ahead of time to tell them about your special needs. If you need assistance with your luggage or boarding the plane, airline personnel will be there to help you. Tell the airline ahead of time of any special dietary needs you have; moreover, the specially prepared meals on a plane are often much better than the regular meals. And be sure to carry your medicines with you, so you can take your pills while you are flying and so your medicines end up exactly where you do. Get up and move about the airplane whenever it's safe to do so (watch out for turbulence, however) to give your joints a little break and stretch your muscles.

Airports can be very hectic, with lots of people rushing between gates, especially during holidays. If possible, plan your trip during a time when not many people are traveling—try to avoid school vacations, for example. And try to fly during times of the day and days of the week when traffic is lighter. Your travel agent can help you with this. Ask your travel agent to recommend travel times that are not holidays at your destination also, so that museums and other sites are less crowded.

If you can, find a flight that travels directly to your destination and doesn't require that you change planes. If you do have to change planes, plan enough time between flights to get to the next gate. The airline will provide a wheelchair or a cart for transportation between gates; try to let them know at the beginning of your trip so the transport will be waiting for you at the interim airport.

Check most of your luggage through to your destination and carry on only what you need (including your medication), so that you are not lugging heavy suitcases around with you. If you use a wheelchair, use the bathroom in the airport before you board the plane. Most bathrooms on planes are very narrow and cannot accommodate a wheelchair.

With these plans all taken care of ahead of time, you should be able to relax and have a wonderful vacation!

My disease has gotten so bad that I think I will soon be unable to work. Will I be eligible for disability benefits?

You may be eligible for disability benefits. The benefits can vary greatly—you may have some coverage from your employer and you may be eligible for other benefits also—and the definition of *disability* can vary. Check with your employer to see if you have short- or long-term disability insurance through work, and check to see how long you have to have been disabled to receive the benefits. Some states have disability programs to which you can contribute through a payroll deduction.

You may also be eligible for Social Security benefits if your arthritis prevents you from being gainfully employed and your condition is expected to last at least one year or to be so severe that it could result in your death. To qualify for Social Security benefits, you will have to undergo an extensive review of your medical history, medical records, and personal physician's reports. You may also have to undergo a comprehensive physical examination. Contact your local Social Security office to learn more about the benefits available in your state.

The Vocational Rehabilitation (VR) program, which is funded by the federal and state governments, is designed to help disabled people become employable. To be eligible for VR, your disability must directly interfere with your ability to work, so you must currently be unemployed to qualify for services. These services include counseling, financial assistance, medical help, education, job training, job placement, and on-the-job assistance. You can find out more about the VR programs in your state by looking under state government services in the phone book.

I'm a veteran of the Korean War. Can I get benefits through the Veterans' Administration system?

All service-related disabilities are covered by the VA, but your arthritis is almost certainly not a result of your service, so you may not be eligible for VA benefits. You might be, though, depending on your income and ability to pay for services, so it's worth contacting your local VA center to find out what benefits you're eligible for.

We are about to change insurance companies and I want to make sure we get a policy with good coverage in case I become disabled. What should I look for?

If you are currently covered by medical insurance, do not drop your policy until you have a new one in place, even if you are not satisfied with it. It's better to have some insurance than none. Check out several different policies before making a decision. But you're right: If you are currently shopping for insurance, you'll want to consider the following:

- Will the policy cover your preexisting condition?

- Will you be able to continue seeing your doctors, or will you have to change?

- Is there a deductible, and can you afford to pay that deductible?

- Are there large copayments for each visit to the doctor?

- After you meet the deductible, what expenses are you responsible for?

- Do low premiums balance out copayments and expenses?

- Is there a cap on the amount you have to pay?

My employer is switching to an HMO, but I have a choice of staying with our old insurance. Will an HMO give me good medical coverage?

HMOs often provide excellent medical care, but they vary greatly. Check on the following things when you are looking at HMOs:

- Check out the list of physicians that the HMO uses. Is your current doctor on the roster? If not, how many of the doctors are accepting new patients?

- Is there a rheumatologist and an orthopedic surgeon experienced in joint surgery on the preferred provider staff? Are these specialists board-certified?

- If you do not find these specialists on the list, contact a representative of the HMO to find out if these services will be covered if your primary-care doctor makes a referral.

- Are you required to use only specific hospitals and physical therapy services? If so, check out the reputations of these providers (your doctor should be able to help) to make sure they are good for people with rheumatoid arthritis.

- Do the primary-care doctors readily refer their patients to specialists? You want to make sure you are going to get all the services you need (rheumatologist, physical and occupational therapists, social worker, etc.) without any difficulty. Some HMOs require authorization from the primary-care doctor for each visit to the specialist. This means you'll have to go back to your primary-care doctor every time you need to see the specialist. And some HMOs have financial incentives for the primary-care doctor *not* to refer patients to specialists.

- If you travel a lot, make sure your HMO will cover emergency care in other states or countries.

- Finally, make sure the HMO is accredited by the National Committee for Quality Assurance (NCQA), which can be reached at (800) 275-7585.

In general, what should I look for in terms of coverage for health insurance or an HMO?

You want to make sure that your policy covers all of the special services you're likely to need, including physical and occupational therapists, a podiatrist, and a clinical psychologist or social worker. A really good policy would also cover alternative services, such as acupuncture and chiropractic treatments (but most do not). Look for a policy that covers the cost of prescription medication as well, because the cost of arthritis medications can be high. Likewise, your policy should cover the cost of assistive devices such as splints, brace, and crutches.

Make sure that your policy will pay for the costs associated with your disease even if it is a preexisting condition. Many carriers are reluctant to take on new patients with chronic medical conditions.

How do I know if I'm eligible for Medicare?

If you are older than 65 or have received Social Security benefits for more than 24 months, you may be eligible for Medicare. Medicare Part A covers inpatient hospital care. The money for Part A comes from the Social Security taxes that are deducted from your paycheck. Medicare Part B covers a percentage of doctors' fees, X rays, and diagnostic tests. You pay a monthly premium for this coverage. Medicare does not pay for medications.

Medicare can help with your medical costs, but it won't pay them all, so you might want to consider getting some additional coverage. Many doctors will not accept a Medicare payment as the full payment for a service, since the Medicare payment is often significantly less than they would receive from private insurance. You also have to pay a large deductible.

What about Medicaid?

Medicaid is available to people with low income, whether or not they are disabled. This program is jointly funded by the federal and state governments. Like Medicare, Medicaid payments to physicians are often lower than private insurance payments, and physicians may be reluctant to treat patients on Medicaid.

Can I deduct my medical expenses from my income taxes?

If you have high medical expenses, you may be able to deduct them. Because of frequent changes in the tax code, you should consult a tax expert. The Internal Revenue Service has several publications that provide information on taxes: #502, *Medical and Dental Expenses*; #524, *Credit for the Elderly or the Disabled*; and #907, *Tax Information for Persons with Handicaps or Disabilities*.

Another option, if your employer offers it, is the cafeteria/flexible benefits program, which allows you to take money out of your paycheck before taxes and set it aside for medical expenses. That way you are not paying taxes on money spent on health care.

I'm afraid I'm going to lose my job if I can't perform up to my old standards. Can I get fired for having arthritis?

The Americans with Disabilities Act (ADA), passed by the U.S. Congress in 1990, bans discrimination against people with disabilities in many areas, including employment. The ADA also protects employers from having to make changes that are unreasonable or expensive (called unreasonable accommodations).

So your employer must make reasonable accommodations to help you keep your job. These include allowing you to shift to a part-time or adjusted work schedule, restructuring your job, providing you with an accessible parking space, providing assistive equipment/devices, providing access to your work site (e.g., a ramp), and/or adjusting the height of your desk.

Your employer does not have to go overboard, though. If the necessary adjustments would represent an undue financial hardship on your employer, your company must give you the choice of sharing in the cost. For example, Chris, a 52-year-old insurance agent, worked in a company with offices on the first and second floors of a small office building. Once he became unable to easily climb the stairs to his second-floor office, he asked his employer to install an elevator. The company looked into the cost and found that they could not afford it, and Chris could not afford to pay any part of it. Chris and the company worked out a great compromise: They moved his office to the first floor, and any meetings he needs to attend are held in the new first-floor conference room, which used to be the library. The library is now on the second floor, so he cannot access books as easily, but his coworkers are happy to help in that regard.

My company is very small. Does the ADA apply to small companies?

The ADA applies to companies that employ 15 or more people. If your company is smaller than that, you cannot use the ADA to help convince your employers to make changes. The ADA applies to private employers, state and local governments, employment agencies, and labor unions. It applies to all aspects of employment, including hiring, job assignments, training, promotion, pay, benefits, and company-sponsored social events.

My wife is becoming progressively disabled and I'd like to work part time for a while until we get adjusted to this new situation. Can my employer fire me for this?

Not if your company has more than 50 employees working within a 75-mile radius and you've worked there for 1,250 hours in the previous 12 months.

The Family and Medical Leave Act (FMLA), which went into effect in August 1993, allows you to take up to three months off from work (unpaid) to care for a spouse, child, or parent who has a serious medical condition. You can take FMLA leave all at one time, over a period of time, or by working part time. The FMLA also allows unpaid leave to care for a newborn, adopted, or foster child, or to care for your own serious medical condition.

When you return to work, you should be able to return to your original or equivalent position, with equivalent pay, benefits, and other terms of employment.

Glossary

Acetaminophen—a drug that relieves pain but does not reduce inflammation.

Acetylcholine—a chemical produced by nerve cells that is important in memory.

Acupuncture—an ancient technique to treat diseases by inserting needles into various parts of the body.

Adrenal glands—small organs located above the kidneys that produce steroid hormones.

Alendronate—a drug used to treat bone loss.

Allopurinol—a drug used to prevent gout attacks by blocking uric acid formation.

Alzheimer's disease—a degenerative disease of the brain characterized by loss of memory.

Amyloid plaques—areas in the brains of patients with Alzheimer's disease where the nerve cells have been destroyed.

Anakinra—an experimental drug for rheumatoid arthritis that blocks the interleukin-1 receptor.

Anemia—a blood condition characterized by a low number of red blood cells.

Angiogenesis—development of new blood vessels.

Angiogenesis inhibitors—drugs that prevent the development of new blood vessels.

Ankylosing spondylitis—an arthritis-like disease that affects the spine, among other joints.

Antibiotics—drugs that kill bacteria.

Anti-inflammatory drugs—drugs that reduce inflammation.

Apoptosis—death of cells by a natural mechanism, also called "programmed cell death."

Arachidonic acid—one of the chemicals in the pathway that produces inflammation.

Arava (leflunomide)—a drug used to slow the progression of rheumatoid arthritis.

Aricept (donepezil hydrochloride)—a drug used to treat Alzheimer's disease.

Arthritis—a disease causing pain, and often inflammation, of the joints. Often also refers to related diseases that cause pain and inflammation in tendons, ligaments, joints, and muscles.

Arthrodesis—a surgical procedure that fuses joint bones together, usually performed to relieve the pain associated with arthritis.

Arthroplasty—a surgical procedure in which the joints are reconstructed using the patient's own tissues as well as artificial joint components. Most arthroplasties involve total joint replacement with natural or artificial materials.

Arthroscopy—examination of the inside of a joint using a fiber-optic instrument inserted through a small incision. Arthroscopy is commonly used in diagnosing and treating sports-related injuries or for performing minor surgical repairs, such as removal of small pieces of torn or loose cartilage.

Arthrotec—a nonsteroidal anti-inflammatory drug (piroxicam) combined with a synthetic prostaglandin (misoprostol). Used to provide pain relief with a lower risk of stomach ulcers than with other NSAIDs.

Aspirin—a commonly used anti-inflammatory and pain reliever.

Autoimmune disease—disease caused by malfunction of the immune system causing it to attack the body's own tissues.

Azathioprine (Imuran)—an immunosuppressive drug used to treat rheumatoid arthritis.

Azulfidine (sulfasalazine)—an antimalarial drug with anti-inflammatory properties used to treat rheumatoid arthritis.

Biologic modifiers—drugs used to treat diseases by modifying the biological process(es) involved in the disease.

Body mechanics—ways of holding and moving the body.

Bunion—inflammation and swelling of the first joint on the big toe.

Bursa—a fibrous sac that acts as a cushion between muscles and bones.

Bursitis—inflammation of the bursa, especially in the shoulder or elbow.

Calcitonin—a drug used to regulate calcium levels in the blood.

Cancer—a group of diseases characterized by uncontrolled growth of cells.

Capsaicin—a chemical that causes a mild burning sensation when applied to the skin, used to distract the brain from other, more serious pain.

Carpal tunnel syndrome—a condition caused by compression of a nerve in the wrist, which causes pain and reduced mobility in the hand.

Cartilage—the tissue that lines the ends of bones, allowing them to slide smoothly without rubbing.

Celebrex (celecoxib)—a COX-2 inhibitor.

Celecoxib (Celebrex)—a COX-2 inhibitor.

Chiropractic therapies—techniques practiced by chiropractors in which the body is manipulated and adjusted to relieve pain.

Chondroitin sulfate—a substance normally found in cartilage and bone.

Cognex (tacrine)—a drug used to treat Alzheimer's disease.

Colchicine—a drug used to treat gout.

Collagen—a protein normally found in cartilage, bone, synovial fluid, and many other tissues in the body.

Computed tomography (CT scan)—a technique for visualizing the inside of the body. A three-dimensional picture is made of various regions of the body.

Corticosteroids—the group of steroid hormones related to cortisone.

Cortisone—a steroid hormone made by the adrenal glands.

COX—*see* Cyclooxygenase.

Cyclooxygenase (COX)—an enzyme found in two forms (COX 1 and COX 2). COX 1 is normally produced by many tissues in the body and is involved in the normal functions of cells. COX 2 is produced in very small amounts in some tissues and in much larger amounts during inflammation. COX 2 is involved in the pathway that produces inflammation.

Cyclooxygenase-2 (COX-2) inhibitors—drugs that stop the enzyme COX 2 from working, thereby reducing inflammation.

Cyclosporine—an immunosuppressive drug used mainly to prevent rejection of transplanted organs.

Cytokines—naturally made chemicals that are used for communication between cells. Many are involved in inflammation.

Cytotec (misoprostol)—a synthetic prostaglandin.

Cytoxan (cyclophosphamide)—an immunosuppressive drug used to treat rheumatoid arthritis.

Degenerative joint disease—osteoarthritis.

Depen (penicillamine)—an immunosuppressive drug used to treat rheumatoid arthritis.

Diclofenac (Voltaren)—a nonsteroidal antiinflammatory drug used to treat pain and inflammation.

Dimethyl sulfoxide (DMSO)—a liquid chemical used by many arthritis patients to relieve pain.

Disease-modifying antirheumatic drugs (DMARDs)—a class of drugs used to treat arthritis by slowing the progression of the disease. Many of these drugs act by impairing the functions of the immune system.

Distal interphalangeal joint (DIP)—the outermost joint on the finger or toe.

Diuretics—drugs that increase the flow of urine.

DMARD—*see* Disease-modifying antirheumatic drugs.

Donepezil hydrochloride (Aricept)—a drug used to treat Alzheimer's disease.

Enbrel (etanercept)—a drug that blocks the cytokine tumor necrosis factor from binding to cells, used to treat rheumatoid arthritis.

Erythrocyte sedimentation rate (ESR)—a blood test used in the diagnosis of rheumatoid arthritis. Measures the rate at which red blood cells fall to the bottom of a tube. This rate is faster in the presence of inflammation.

Etanercept (Enbrel)—a drug that blocks the cytokine tumor necrosis factor from binding to cells, used to treat rheumatoid arthritis.

Etidronate—a drug used to treat bone loss.

Extra-articular manifestations of rheumatoid arthritis—symptoms that occur outside of the joints, such as vasculitis and ophthalmitis.

Feldene (piroxicam)—a nonsteroidal anti-inflammatory drug.

Felty's syndrome—a condition that affects the blood, sometimes found in people with rheumatoid arthritis.

Fibromyalgia—a disease involving pain in muscles or joints with no clinical signs of inflammation. Linked to stress.

5-Fluorouracil (5-FU)—a drug used to treat cancer.

Flare-ups—periods during which the symptoms of disease get worse.

Free radicals—atoms that can cause chemical reactions. Involved in inflammation and other disease conditions.

Genetic predisposition—the tendency, because of one's genetic makeup, to develop a disease.

Glucosamine—a chemical normally found in many tissues.

Gout—an arthritis-like disease characterized by painful joints.

Hereditary predisposition—*see* Genetic predisposition.

HLA-DR4—a marker in the genes found in some people with rheumatoid arthritis.

Homeopathy—an alternative medical practice that treats diseases by administration of a minute amount of substances that would produce symptoms of the disease in a healthy person.

Hormone replacement therapy—treatment of menopause with estrogen.

Hyaluron—a substance normally found in synovial fluid and other viscous fluids in the body.

Hydrotherapy—exercise and physical therapy performed in warm water.

Hydroxychloroquine (Plaquenil)—an antimalarial drug used to treat rheumatic arthritis.

Ibuprofen—a nonsteroidal anti-inflammatory drug used to treat pain and inflammation.

Immune system—the system of cells and chemicals in the body that fights diseases.

Immunosuppressive drugs—drugs that decrease the immune response.

Imuran (azathioprine)—an immunosuppressive drug used to treat rheumatoid arthritis.

Indocin (indomethacin)—a nonsteroidal anti-inflammatory drug used to treat pain and inflammation.

Indomethacin (Indocin)—a nonsteroidal anti-inflammatory drug used to treat pain and inflammation.

Inflammation—a reaction to injury or infection resulting in redness, heat, swelling, pain, and loss of function in the affected areas.

Infliximab (Remicade)—an experimental drug used to treat rheumatoid arthritis by blocking the cytokine interleukin-1.

Interleukin-1 (IL-1)—a cytokine involved in inflammation.

Interphalangeal joints (IP)—the joints of the fingers.

Isometric exercise—a type of exercise that uses resistance to build muscle strength.

Isotonic exercise—a type of exercise that does not use resistance, but still builds muscle strength.

Joint—the structure in the body where two bones come together.

Juvenile rheumatoid arthritis—a form of rheumatoid arthritis found in children.

Leflunomide (Arava)—a drug used to treat rheumatoid arthritis.

Leucovorin—a drug used to treat cancer.

Leukotriene inhibitors—drugs that prevent the formation of leukotriene.

Leukotrienes—a group of chemicals produced during inflammation and allergic responses.

Ligaments—thick, cordlike fibers anchored to bones to keep them correctly lined up.

Lumbago—a painful inflammation of the muscles in the lower back.

Lupus erythematosus—an autoimmune, arthritis-like disease characterized by painful joints and inflammation of the skin.

Lyme disease—a joint infection caused by bacteria transmitted by a tick. Characterized by widespread joint pain.

Magnetic resonance imaging (MRI)—a technique used to visualize the inside of the body. Produces computerized images of various body organs.

Meloxicam—a nonsteroidal anti-inflammatory agent that acts preferentially on COX 2.

Metacarpophalangeal joint (MCP)—the joint where the finger meets the hand.

Metatarsophalangeal joint—joint on the toe.

Methotrexate—a powerful drug used to treat rheumatoid arthritis and many types of cancer.

Minocin (minocycline)—an antibiotic that has shown some efficacy in treating rheumatoid arthritis.

Minocycline (Minocin)—an antibiotic that has shown some efficacy in treating rheumatoid arthritis.

Misoprostol (Cytotoc)—a synthetic prostaglandin.

Naproxen—a nonsteroidal anti-inflammatory agent.

Neoplasia—the process of tumor formation.

Neoral (cyclosporine)—an immunosuppressive drug used mainly to prevent rejection of transplanted organs.

Nitric oxide—a chemical produced during inflammation.

Nitro-NSAIDs—nonsteroidal anti-inflammatory drugs coupled to nitric oxide.

Nodule—an accumulation of inflammatory tissue under the skin. The presence of nodules may indicate more serious disease.

Nonacetylated salicylates—aspirin-like drugs that are easier on the stomach.

Nonsteroidal anti-inflammatory drugs (NSAIDs)—a group of drugs that act to reduce pain and inflammation by inhibiting the action of the COX enzymes.

NSAID—*see* Nonsteroidal anti-inflammatory drugs.

Occupational therapy—therapy that evaluates the impact of disease on daily activities at home and on the job. An occupational therapist can help the patient figure out ways to perform tasks to put less stress on the joints.

Omega-3 fatty acids—a group of chemicals found in large amounts in certain foods.

Ophthalmitis—inflammation of the eyes found in some cases of rheumatoid arthritis.

Oral medication—medication that can be taken by mouth rather than by injection.

Orthopedic surgeon—a surgeon who works on bones.

Osteoarthritis—the most common form of arthritis, also known as degenerative arthritis or degenerative joint disease. Caused by changes in the cartilage, possibly from wear and tear on the joint over time.

Osteoporosis—a condition caused by thinning of the bones, resulting in increased likelihood of fractures.

Osteotomy—a surgical procedure during which the bone is removed to allow realignment to a better position.

Penicillamine (Cuprimine, Depen)—an immunosuppressive drug used to treat rheumatoid arthritis.

Physical therapy—therapy designed to help with the physical aspects of an illness and to design exercise programs.

Piroxicam (Feldene)—a nonsteroidal anti-inflammatory agent.

Placebo—a medication that has no known effect on the disease for which it is being used. Used in clinical trials as comparison with drugs being tested.

Plaquenil (hydroxychloroquine)—an antimalarial drug used to treat rheumatoid arthritis.

Platelets—blood components involved in blood clotting.

Podiatrist—a specialist in the care and treatment of the human foot.

Prednisone—a corticosteroid.

Propranolol—a beta blocker used to treat abnormal heart rhythms and angina.

Prostaglandins—a group of naturally occurring chemicals involved in inflammation, as well as other processes in the body.

Proteoglycans—a group of chemicals commonly found in connective tissue in the body.

Proximal interphalangeal joint (PIP)—the middle joint on the finger or toe.

Range of motion—the range of movement that a joint can make. Used to measure the severity of the arthritis. Also refers to a type of exercise.

Remicade (infliximab)—an experimental drug to treat rheumatoid arthritis by blocking the cytokine interleukin-1.

Remission—a period during which the symptoms of the disease disappear.

Rheumatoid arthritis—an autoimmune type of arthritis characterized by pain and swelling in the joints.

Rheumatoid factor—a substance found in large amounts in some people with rheumatoid arthritis. Its presence is useful as a diagnostic tool.

Rheumatoid lung—a condition characterized by inflammation of the lung. Found in some patients with severe rheumatoid arthritis.

Rheumatoid nodules—an accumulation of inflammatory tissue under the skin. The presence of nodules may indicate more serious disease.

Rheumatologist—a physician who specializes in the diagnosis and treatment of arthritis and related diseases.

Rofecoxib (Vioxx)—a COX-2 inhibitor.

Salicylates—aspirinlike drugs.

Sciatica—inflammation of the sciatic nerve, causing pain in the lower back and leg.

Scleroderma—an arthritis-like disease characterized by thickening of the skin.

Selegiline—a drug used to treat Parkinson's disease.

Slow-acting drugs—*see* Disease-modifying antirheumatic drugs.

Splints—devices used to support the joints.

Steroids—*see* Corticosteroids.

Stomach ulcer—painful stomach condition caused by erosion of the lining of the stomach.

Synovectomy—surgical removal of the synovium or joint lining.

Synovial fluid—a clear, viscous fluid produced by the synovium that fills the joint space and acts as a lubricant.

Synovium—the membrane that lines the inside of the joint.

Systemic illness—illness throughout the entire body.

Tacrine (Cognex)—a drug used to treat Alzheimer's disease.

Tendonitis—inflammation of the tendons.

Tendons—strong bands of tissue that connect bones to muscles.

Thalidomide—a powerful drug used to treat leprosy and being investigated as a drug to treat cancer.

Theophylline—a bronchodilator used to treat asthma.

Topical analgesics—pain-killing creams rubbed on the skin.

Toxicity—a measure of the seriousness of the side effects produced by a drug.

Tumor necrosis factor (TNF)—a cytokine involved in many cellular processes, including inflammation.

Uric acid—a waste product of cellular processes, normally found in small amounts in blood. Found in larger amounts in the synovial fluid of patients with gout.

Vasculitis—inflammation of the lining of the blood vessels.

Vertebrae—bones making up the spine.

Vioxx (rofecoxib)—a COX-2 inhibitor.

Voltaren (diclofenac)—a nonsteroidal anti-inflammatory drug.

Warfarin—a blood-thinning drug used to reduce the risk of heart attack or stroke.

Zileuton (Zyflo)—a drug that decreases the production of leukotrienes. Used in the treatment of asthma.

∾

Resources

∾ **Books on Rheumatoid Arthritis for Adults**

The following list includes books on the causes of and treatments for rheumatoid arthritis, as well as exercises and diets that may help relieve the pain.

All About Arthritis: Past, Present, and Future. Derrick Brewerton (Harvard University Press) 1995.

Arthritis (Health Watch). Susan Dudley Gold, Brian J. Keroack (Crestwood House) 1997.

Arthritis (Your Personal Health Series). John Thompson, Robert F. Meenan (Key Porter Books) 1996.

Arthritis Alternatives. Irna and Laurence Gold (Facts on File Publications) 1985.

Arthritis and Chinese Herbal Medicine. Pi-Kwang

Tsung, Hong-Ven Hsu (Oriental Healing Arts Institute) 1993.

Arthritis and Common Sense. Dale Alexander, H. E. Kirschner (Simon & Schuster) 1981.

Arthritis and Folk Medicine. D. C. Jarvis (Fawcett Books) 1991.

Arthritis: A Take-Care-of-Yourself Health Guide for Understanding Your Arthritis. James F. Fries (Perseus Press) 1995.

Arthritis Begone!: A Doctor's Rx for Easy, Safe, Inexpensive—and Effective—Treatments for Your Arthritis Pain. John B. Irwin (Keats Publishing) 1997.

Arthritis Breakthrough. Henry Scammell, Thomas Brown McPherson (M. Evans) 1993.

The Arthritis Cure. Jason Theodosakis, Brenda Adderly, Barry Fox (Griffin Trade Paperback), 1997.

The Arthritis Cure Cookbook. Lissa De Angelis, Brenda D. Adderly (National Book Network) 1998.

The Arthritis Exercise Book: Gentle, Joint-by-Joint Exercises to Keep You Flexible and Independent. Gwen Ellert, Barry Koehler (NTC/Contemporary Publishing) 1990.

Arthritis Handbook. Theodore Rooney, Patty Rooney (Ballantine Books) 1990.

The Arthritis Healthy Exchanges Cookbook. Joanna M. Lund (Perigee) 1998.

The Arthritis Helpbook: A Tested, Self-Management Program for Coping with Arthritis and Fibromyalgia. Kate Lorig, James F. Fries (Perseus Press) 1995.

The Arthritis Helpbook: A Tested, Self-Management Program for Coping with Your Arthritis. Kate Lorig, James F. Fries (Addison-Wesley) 1990.

Arthritis of the Hip and Knee: The Active Person's Guide to Taking Charge. Ronald J. Allen, S. David

Stulberg, Victoria Anne Brander, Pat Lee (Peachtree Publishers) 1998.

Arthritis 101. Questions You Have. Answers You Need. An official publication of the Arthritis Foundation (Longstreet Press) 1997.

Arthritis Relief: Breakthroughs in Natural Healing. Deborah L. Wilcox (Rhodes & Easton) 1997.

The Arthritis Solution. Larry Katzenstein, Winifred Conkling (Signet) 1997.

The Arthritis Solution. David B. Sudderth, Joseph Kandel (Prima Publishing) 1997.

Arthritis: Sound Techniques for Healing (audio cassette). Robert Friedman, Kelly Howell (Brain Sync Corp.) 1993.

The Arthritis Sourcebook. Kathy Cochran Angel, Earl J. Brewer, Jr. (Lowell House) 1998.

Arthritis: Stop Suffering, Start Moving. Darlene Cohen (Walker Publishing) 1995.

Arthritis: The Chinese Way of Healing and Prevention. Jwing-Ming Yang (Ymaa Publications) 1997.

Arthritis: What Exercises Work. David Sobel, Arthur C. Klein, John Bland (St. Martin's Press) 1995.

Arthritis: What Works. David Sobel, Arthur C. Klein, Willibald Nagler (St. Martin's Press) 1992.

Arthritis: Your Complete Exercise Guide (Cooper Clinic and Research Institute Fitness Series). Neil F. Gordon (Human Kinetics Publishing) 1992.

The Columbia Presbyterian Osteoarthritis Handbook: The Complete Guide to the Most Common Form of Arthritis. Suzanne Loebl, Ronald P. Grelsamer (Macmillan General Reference) 1997.

Coping with Rheumatoid Arthritis. Robert H. Phillips (Avery) 1988.

A Doctor's New Proven Home Cure for Arthritis. Giraud

W. Campbell, Robert B. Stone (Prentice Hall Trade) 1989.

The Duke University Medical Center Book of Arthritis. David S. Pisetsky, Susan Flamholtz Trien (Ballantine Books) 1992.

The Essential Arthritis Cookbook: Kitchen Basics for People with Arthritis, Fibromyalgia, and other Chronic Pain and Fatigue. Sarah L. Morgan, Linda Hachfeld (Appletree Press) 1995.

Exercise and Arthritis: A Guide to Pain-Free Movement. Margaret Hills, Janet Horwood (Peoples Medical Society) 1997.

Exercise Beats Arthritis: An Easy-to-Follow Program of Exercises. Valerie Sayce, Ian Fraser (Bull Publishing) 1998.

50 Ways to Cope with Arthritis. Diana L. Anderson (Signet) 1996.

Gentle Relaxing and Strengthening Movements for People with Back Problems, Arthritis, and MS. Ruth Bender (Ruben Publishing) 1983.

Gentle Yoga for People with Arthritis, Stroke Damage, Multiple Sclerosis, and in Wheelchairs. Loena Belland, Eudora Seyfer, Lorna Bell (Gentle Yoga) 1990.

Health Journeys for People with Rheumatoid Arthritis or Lupus. Belleruth Naperstek (Health Journeys) 1994.

How to Eat Away Arthritis. Lauri M. Aesoph (Prentice Hall) 1996.

Living with Arthritis. John Shenkman (Franklin Watts) 1990.

Living with Arthritis: Successful Strategies to Help Manage the Pain and Remain Active. Harry Shen, Cheryl Solimini, Kent Humphreys (Plume) 1993.

Living with Rheumatoid Arthritis. Tammi L Shlotzhauer

and James L. McGuire (The Johns Hopkins University Press) 1993.

Maximizing the Arthritis Cure: A Step-by-Step Program to Faster, Stronger Healing During Any Stage of the Cure. Jason Theodosakis, Barry Fox, Sam Tsoutsouvas, Brenda D. Adderly (St. Martin's Press) 1998.

Mechanisms and Models in Rheumatoid Arthritis. E. R. Pettipher, Brian Henderson, Jo Edwards, John A. Edwards (Academic Press) 1995.

Natural Medicine for Arthritis (The Dell Natural Medicine Library). Winifred Conkling, Lynn Sonberg (Dell Books) 1997.

Natural Medicine for Arthritis: The Best Alternative Methods for Relieving Pain and Stiffness, from Food and Herbs to Acupuncture and Homeopathy. Glenn S. Rothfeld, Suzanne LeVert (Rodale Press) 1996.

Natural Relief for Arthritis. Carol Keough (Rodale Press) 1983.

The New Arthritis Breakthrough. Henry Scammell (M. Evans) 1993.

The New Arthritis Relief Diet: Proven Steps to Stop Inflammation, Prevent Joint Damage, Decrease Medication, and Improve the Quality of Your Life. James Scala (Plume) 1998.

Primer on the Rheumatic Diseases: An Official Publication of the Arthritis Foundation. Cornelia M. Weyand, Robert Wortmann, John H. Klippel (Andrews & McMeel) 1998.

Recipes for Health. Arthritis and Rheumatism: Delicious Recipes to Relieve the Symptoms of Arthritis and Rheumatism. Alkmini Chaitow, Leon Chaitow (Thorsons Publishing) 1998.

Taking Control of Arthritis (Thorndike Large Print Self-

Help Specials). Fred G. Kantrowitz (Thorndike Press) 1992.

Textbook of Rheumatology. William N. Kelley, Edward D. Harris, Shaun Ruddy (W. B. Saunders) 1997.

Toward Healthy Living: A Wellness Journal. The Arthritis Foundation (Longstreet Press) 1998.

Treating Arthritis, Carpal Tunnel Syndrome, and Joint Conditions (Physicians' Guides to Healing, No. 2). Alan Pressman, Herbert D. Goodman, Karen Lane, Philip Lief Group (Berkley Publishing Group) 1997.

250 Tips for Making Life with Arthritis Easier. Shelley Peterman Schwarz (Longstreet Press) 1997.

Understanding Arthritis. What It Is, How to Treat It, How to Cope with It. The Arthritis Foundation (Macmillan General Reference) 1986.

Why Arthritis? Searching for the Cause and Cure of Rheumatoid Disease. Harold W. Clark, Karen L. Jacob (Avelrod Publishing) 1997.

Winning with Arthritis. Harris H. McIlwain, Joel C. Silverfield, Michael C. Burnette, Debra Bruce (John Wiley & Sons) 1997.

❧ Books for Children and Families of Children with Juvenile Rheumatoid Arthritis

Life can be difficult for a child with arthritis. The good books listed below may help the child and family cope with this disease.

Nicole's Story: A Book About a Girl with Juvenile Rheumatoid Arthritis. Virginia Tortorica Aldape, Lillian S. Kossacoff (Lemer Publications) 1996.

Parenting a Child with Arthritis: A Practical, Empathetic Guide to Help You and Your Child Live with Arthritis. Kathy Cochran Angel, Earl J. Brewer, Jr., C. Everett Koop (Lowell House) 1992.

Raising a Child with Arthritis: Parent's Guide. Arthritis Foundation (Longstreet Press) 1998.

Your Child with Arthritis: A Family Guide to Caregiving. Lori B. Tucker, Bethany A. Denardo, Judith A. Stebulis, Jane G. Schaller (Johns Hopkins University Press) 1996.

∾ Arthritis and Disability-Related Websites and Homepages on the Internet

ABLEDATA (http://www.abledata.com)

ABLEDATA is a federally funded project that provides information on assistive technology and disability-related products. The ABLEDATA database contains information on 17,000 currently available products. ABLEDATA also publishes fact sheets and consumer guides and can also be reached at (800) 227-0216.

About.com Guide to Arthritis (http://arthritis.about.com)

Provides a wealth of information through links to several excellent sites for information on the disease, diagnosis, current treatments, and drugs under development. Also provides a bulletin board, chat room, and newsletter.

American Academy of Physical Medicine and Rehabilitation (http://www.aapmr.org)

The AAPMR is the national society of physicians

who are specialists in the field of physical medicine and rehabilitation. They are called physiatrists. Physiatrists work with patients who have chronic pain, such as that caused by arthritis, and those with spinal cord injuries or other debilitating conditions. This website can help you find a physiatrist in your area.

American College of Rheumatology
(http://www.rheumatology.org)

Contains information on research, education, new treatments, etc. Links to press releases on new information.

American Physical Therapy Association
(http://www.apta.org)

The APTA is a professional organization of physical therapists. This website contains mostly information for professionals but also provides information on how to get some patient-oriented booklets.

Arthritis Bookstore (http://mediconsult.com/arthritis/ store/books/)

Provides a list and description of books that would be of interest to people with arthritis and their families.

Arthritis Foundation
(http://www.arthritis.org)

The official website of the Arthritis Foundation. Provides information on the disease and resources available to patients and families. Lots of patient-oriented tips and information on how to contact your local chapter of the Arthritis Foundation. Preview of and subscription information for *Arthritis Today,* the official magazine of the Arthritis Foundation.

**Arthritis: Mediconsult.com
(http://mediconsult.com/arthritis)**
Provides educational material, drug information, and clinical trial updates.

**The Design Linc. Accessibility Design Resources
(http://www.designlinc.com/designlinc/organiz.htm)**
Provides addresses and phone numbers listed by state for groups that provide resources to people with disabilities.

**Fact Sheet on Rheumatoid Arthritis
(http://www.rheumatology.org/patient/ra.htm)**
Provides basic information on the disease, diagnosis, and treatment.

**Handilinks to Sports Disabilities
(http://www.ahandyguide.com/cat1/d/d341.htm)**
Provides links to many websites with information on sports activities for the disabled.

National Institute of Arthritis and Musculoskeletal and Skin Diseases (http://www.nih.gov/niams)
Provides information on research that is being conducted in arthritis and related diseases.

National Institute on Disability and Rehabilitation Research (http://www.ed.gov/offices/OSERS/NIDRR)
Provides up-to-date information on assistive technology and other disability issues.

**National Rehabilitation Information Center
(http://www.naric.com/naric)**
Provides the results of federally funded research proj-

ects and listings of other available literature on disabilities and rehabilitation.

New York Online Access to Health
(http://www.noah.cuny.edu)

An easy-to-use health information vehicle for consumers. Available in English and Spanish.

Stanford University Rheumatology Department
(http://www.stanford.edu/group/rheum/
rheuhome.html)

Provides information on clinical trials of new drugs to treat rheumatoid arthritis. Also has information on the ARAMIS 2000 long-term survey of outcomes in arthritis.

∾ Support and Networking Organizations and Associations

ARTHRITIS ORGANIZATIONS

The Arthritis Foundation, American Juvenile Arthritis Organization, and the National Institute of Arthritis and Musculoskeletal and Skin Diseases are three of the main organizations for information about arthritis.

The Arthritis Foundation
1330 West Peachtree Street
Atlanta, GA 30309
(800) 283-7800
(404) 872-7100
http://www.arthritis.org

If you want more information on rheumatoid arthritis or any other form of arthritis, contact the Arthritis Foundation. The Arthritis Foundation was formed in 1948 and is the leading national organization devoted to promoting education and research on all forms of arthritis. The Foundation is a source of help and hope for nearly 40 million Americans who have arthritis and related conditions. Through the Foundation, you can obtain literature with information about the disease, join patient support groups, use the lending library, and attend lectures. Many helpful brochures are available free of charge from the Foundation (see page 210). Local chapters raise funds to train doctors and researchers to investigate the causes, treatment, and prevention of arthritis and related diseases.

American Juvenile Arthritis Organization
1330 West Peachtree Street
Atlanta, GA 30309
(800) 283-7800
(404) 872-7100
http://www.arthritis.org/ajao/

The American Juvenile Arthritis Organization (AJAO) is composed of children, parents, teachers, and others concerned specifically with juvenile arthritis.

The National Institute of Arthritis and Musculoskeletal and Skin Diseases
Building 31, Room 4C05
31 Center Drive
MSC 2350
Bethesda, MD 20892-2350

(301) 907-8900
http://www.nih.gov/niams

The National Institute of Arthritis and Musculoskeletal and Skin Diseases has publications and tapes and provides information about community services.

OTHER ORGANIZATIONS

The following organizations provide services and educational material on arthritis and related diseases.

Natural Health Practitioners

American Association of Oriental Medicine
433 Front Street
Capasauqua, PA 18032
(610) 433-2448
http://www.aaom.org

American Chiropractic Association
1701 Clarendon Boulevard
Arlington, VA 22209
(800) 986-4636
http://www.amerchiro.org

American Holistic Medicine Association
6728 Old McLean Village Drive
McLean, VA 22101
(703) 556-9728
http://www.holisticmedicine.org

National Center for Homeopathy
801 North Fairfax

Suite 306
Alexandria, VA 22314
(703) 548-7790
http://www.healthy.net/nch/

Physical Therapy

American Academy of Physical Medicine and Rehabilitation
One IBM Plaza
Chicago, IL 60611-3604
(312) 464-9700
http://www.aapmr.org

American Physical Therapy Association
1156 15th Street, NW
Washington, DC 20005
(703) 706-3248
http://www.apta.org

National Rehabilitation Information Center
8455 Colsville Road
Suite 935
Silver Spring, MD 20910-3319
(800) 346-2742
http://www.naric.com/naric

Ankylosing Spondylitis

Spondylitis Association of America
14827 Ventura Boulevard
Suite 222
P.O. Box 5872

Sherman Oaks, CA 91413
(800) 777-8189

Fibromyalgia

American Chronic Pain Association
P.O. Box 850
Rocklin, CA 95677
(916) 632-0922
http://www.theacpa.org

The Fibromyalgia Alliance of America
P.O. Box 21990
Columbus, OH 43221-0990
(614) 457-4222

The Fibromyalgia Network
P.O. Box 31750
Tucson, AZ 85751-1750
(800) 853-2929
http://www.fmnetnews.com

National Chronic Fatigue Syndrome and Fibromyalgia Association
3521 Broadway
Suite 222
P.O. Box 18426
Kansas City, MO 64133
(816) 931-4777

Lupus Erythematosus

Lupus Foundation of America
1300 Picard Drive
Suite 200

Rockville, MD 20850-4303
(800) 558-0121
(301) 670-9292
http://internet-plaza.net/lupus

Scleroderma

Scleroderma Foundation
89 Newbury Street
Danvers, MA 01923
(978) 750-4499
http://www.scleroderma.org

Scleroderma International Foundation
704 Gardner Center Road
New Castle, PA 16101
(724) 652-3109

Scleroderma Research Foundation
Pueblo Medical Commons
2320 Bath Street
Suite 307
Santa Barbara, CA 93105
(800) 441-CURE
http://www.srfcure.org

Sjogren's Syndrome

National Sjogren's Syndrome Foundation
3201 West Evans Drive
Phoenix, AZ 85023
(800) 395-6772
http://www.sjogrens.org

Sjogren's Syndrome Foundation
333 North Broadway
Jericho, NY 11753
(800) 4-SJOGREN
http://www.sjogrens.com

RESOURCES FOR OUTDOOR ACTIVITIES

The following resources specialize in information and products for outdoor activities:

Buckmasters Disabled Chapter
Call David Sullivan, (205) 339-2800

Provides services for disabled whitetail deer hunters.

Fishing Has No Boundaries, Inc.
P.O. Box 175
Hayward, WI 54843
(800) 243-3462
(715) 634-3185

Florida Disabled Outdoors Association
2213 Tallahassee Drive
Tallahassee, FL 32308
David Jones, (850) 668-7323

Statewide organization dedicated to promoting and supporting recreation opportunities and outdoor activities for disabled sportsmen.

Freedom Rider
P.O. Box 4188
Dedham, MA 02027-4188
(888) 253-8811

A catalog of products to assist the disabled with horseback riding.

Shake-a-Leg
2600 Bayshore Drive
Miami, FL 33133
(305) 858-5550

Offers sailing trips with rehabilitation.

∾ Professional Organizations

Professional organizations can help you find a health-care provider in your area.

American College of Rheumatology
1800 Century Place, Suite 250
Atlanta, GA 30345
(404) 633-3777
http://www.rheumatology.org

If you want to find a rheumatologist in your area, try contacting the American College of Rheumatology (ACR). The ACR is a professional organization for rheumatologists that sponsors a meeting every year at which new research and treatment results are presented.

American Occupational Therapy Association
4720 Montgomery Lane
P.O. Box 31220
Bethesda, MD 20824-1220
(800) 729-2682
http://www.aota.org

The American Occupational Therapy Association (AOTA) is the professional group for occupational therapists. The members of this association provide services to people whose lives have been disrupted by physical injury or illness or by the aging process. The AOTA can help you find an occupational therapist in your area.

American Physical Therapy Association
1156 15th Street, NW
Washington, DC 20005
(703) 706-3248
http://www.apta.org

The American Physical Therapy Association (APTA) is a national professional group representing more than 75,000 physical therapists. The goal of the APTA is to foster advances in physical therapy practice, research, and education. To obtain a list of physical therapists in your area, contact the APTA.

National Association for Home Care
228 7th Street, SE
Washington, DC 20003
(202) 547-7424

The National Association for Home Care (NAHC) represents home-care professionals. Members of this organization meet standards set by the NAHC.

National Rehabilitation Association
633 South Washington Street
Alexandria, VA 22314
(703) 836-0850
http://www.nationalrehab.org

The National Rehabilitation Association (NRA) is comprised of physicians, therapists of all kinds, counselors, and other practitioners who work with the physically disabled.

∾ Arthritis Magazines, Newsletters, and Brochures

MAGAZINES

Accent on Living
P.O. Box 700
Bloomington, IL 61702
(309) 378-2961
http://www.accentonliving.com

Accent on Living provides a quarterly publication and books and videos for people with disabilities.

Arthritis Today
The Arthritis Foundation
1330 West Peachtree Street
Atlanta, GA 30309
(800) 283-7800
(404) 872-7100
http://www.arthritis.org

Arthritis Today is published six times a year by the Arthritis Foundation and is the main magazine for people with arthritis.

***Pelaestra: Forum of Sport, Physical Education &
Recreation for Those with Disabilities***
P.O. Box 508
Macomb, IL 61455
(309) 833-1902
http://www.pelaestra.com

This magazine, now in its fifteenth year, is a quarterly
publication for all individuals interested in sports, physical education, and recreation involving people with disabilities.

WE Magazine
495 Broadway
New York, NY 10012
(800) WEMAG 26
http://www.wemagazine.com

WE magazine is a lifestyle magazine for people with
disabilities. The website also provides a variety of services and information on products for the disabled.

ARTHRITIS FOUNDATION BROCHURES

Many excellent brochures on rheumatoid arthritis are
available from the Arthritis Foundation. To locate your
local chapter of the foundation, call toll-free (800) 283-
7800. To order pamphlets from the foundation, write to
The Arthritis Foundation, P.O. Box 19000, Atlanta, GA
30326. The following is a listing of some of the brochures available:

Arthritis and Employment provides information on how to function successfully at work.

Arthritis Answers is an overview of the common types of arthritis and related conditions, including treatments.

Arthritis Guide to Insurance for People with Arthritis helps you understand insurance coverage for arthritis-related treatments.

Arthritis in the Workplace provides information to consider when choosing a career, plus interviewing tips and ways to make your workspace more arthritis-friendly.

Choosing a Health Plan contains tips on how to obtain medical coverage and explanations of different types of health plans.

Exercise and Your Arthritis provides tips on how to exercise better.

A Guide to Intimacy with Arthritis talks about arthritis and physical intimacy.

Guide to Social Security Disability Insurance for People with Arthritis.

Managing Your Activities contains suggestions on how to use your joints wisely during daily activities, plus lists of self-help aids.

Managing Your Fatigue provides basic information about arthritis-related fatigue and tips on how to manage it.

Managing Your Health Care provides tips on establishing and strengthening communication with your doctor.

Managing Your Pain is an overview of how arthritis causes pain, how the body reacts to pain, and how you can manage it.

Managing Your Stress contains tips on how to reduce the stress associated with arthritis.

Rheumatoid Arthritis provides information on the disease.

Travel Tips for People with Arthritis.

Understanding Arthritis in African Americans is an overview of the arthritis-related conditions that are more likely to affect African Americans.

GOVERNMENT PUBLICATIONS

Consumer Information Catalog, available from the Consumer Information Center, Pueblo, CO 81009, is a catalog of free and low-cost federal publications on many topics, including federal benefits and health issues. This free catalog is an excellent resource.

Disability, available from your local Social Security office (or call the Social Security toll-free hotline at (800) 234-5772), provides information on disability benefits.

Medicare, available from your local Social Security office (or call the Social Security toll-free hotline at (800) 234-5772), is a guide to Medicare benefits.

Medicaid. For more information on Medicaid, write to the Health Care Financing Administration, Inquiries Staff, Room GF-3, East Lowrise Building, Baltimore, MD 21207.

Nutrition and Your Health: Dietary Guidelines for Americans, available from the U.S. Department of Agriculture (202-205-8333) and U.S. Department of Health and Human Services (202-619-0257). This pamphlet can be ordered from the Consumer Information Catalog, Consumer Information Center, Pueblo, CO 81009.

Pocket Guide to Federal Help for Individuals with Disabilities, available from the U.S. Department of Education (Ed. Pubs. 8242, Sandy Court, Jessup, MD 20794) is a guide to federal money available for people with disabilities. (877) 433-7827.

Supplemental Security Income, available from your local Social Security office (or call the Social Security toll-free hotline at (800) 234-5772), is a guide to Social Security benefits.

Traveling with a Disability. A list of guides for handicapped travelers can be obtained from the President's Committee on Employment of People with Disabilities, 1111 20th St. NW, Washington, DC 20210. (202) 376-6200.

Understanding Social Security, available from your local Social Security office (or call the Social Security toll-free hotline at (800) 234-5772), helps you understand your Social Security benefits.

Working While Disabled . . . How Social Security Can Help, available from your local Social Security office (or call the Social Security toll-free hotline at (800) 234-5772), provides information on working with a disability and your supplemental Social Security benefits.

ADDITIONAL BROCHURES AND DIRECTORIES ON TRAVEL

Directory of Travel Agencies for the Disabled, by Helen Hecker, R.N., is available from Twin Peaks Press, P.O. Box 129, Vancouver, WA 98666-0129. (800) 637-2256.

How to Travel with Arthritis is an on-line brochure available from the Society for the Advancement of Travel for the Handicapped (SATH), 347 Fifth Avenue, New York, NY 10016. (212) 447-0027; *http://www.sath.org*.

Travel for the Disabled: A Handbook of Travel Resources and 500 Worldwide Access Guides, by Helen Hecker, R.N., is also available from Twin Peaks Press.

∾ Services

THE ARTHRITIS FOUNDATION

The Arthritis Foundation offers several courses and programs for people with arthritis. Contact your local Arthritis Foundation office to find out if any of the following services are offered in your area. These programs are designed to help you live a happy, healthy, and fulfilling life despite your disease. Some are designed to help you live more independently and perform your daily tasks without endangering your joints. Others are exercise programs—exercising makes you more fit and healthy, keeps your bones and muscles strong, gives you energy, and helps you feel better overall—designed specifically for those with arthritis.

* *Arthritis Self-Help Course.* Learn how to take control of your own care and be more independent and safer in this six-week (15-hour) class for people with arthritis.

* *Warm-Water Exercise Program.* This is a 6- to 10-week exercise program in a heated pool, designed especially for people with joint disease.

- *Land exercise programs.* Exercise classes are offered at a variety of levels, where you will learn to move more easily. You can also purchase a videotape and exercise at home.

- *Support groups and clubs.* It can be very useful to share your stories—the successes and challenges—with others in the same boat. Through support groups you can also get tips on how to overcome some problems associated with arthritis.

NATIONAL COMMITTEE FOR QUALITY ASSURANCE (NCQA)

To check whether your HMO is accredited, contact the National Committee for Quality Assurance (NCQA), which can be reached at (800) 275-7585.

MEDIC ALERT

For more information about obtaining a Medic Alert bracelet, which will identify you as having rheumatoid arthritis, write to Medic Alert, Box 1009, Turlock, CA 95380 or call (800) 825-3785.

∾ Instructional Videotapes

Several excellent videotapes are available demonstrating exercises for people with arthritis.

- *People with Arthritis Can Exercise (PACE)* is a program that incorporates flexibility, strengthening, and endurance exercises. For information on the PACE programs, write to the Arthritis Foundation, P.O. Box 1616, Alpharetta, GA 30009, or call (800) 207-8633.

- *Feeling Good with Arthritis* videotapes. Xenejenex, 10 Tower Office Park, Suite 420, Woburn, MA 01801. (781) 938-9922.

- *PEP (Pool Exercise Program)* videotape. Codeveloped by the YMCA and the Arthritis Foundation, this water exercise program helps relieve the strain on muscles and joints. The videotape shows you how to exercise on your own. For information on the PACE programs, write to the Arthritis Foundation, PEP Order Center, P.O. Box 1616, Alpharetta, GA 30009, or call (800) 207-8633

≈

Bibliography

≈ **CHAPTER ONE**

The Arthritis Foundation, *Arthritis 101*, Marietta, GA: Longstreet Press, 1997.

The Arthritis Foundation, *Rheumatoid Arthritis*, Arthritis Foundation brochure.

Bunker, V. W., "The role of nutrition in osteoporosis," *British Journal of Biomedical Science*, 51: 228–240, 1994.

Edwards, J., *Notes on Rheumatology*, Welwyn Garden City, UK: Broadwater Press, Ltd., 1991.

Gremillion, R. B., van Vollenhoven, R. F. "Rheumatoid arthritis," *Post Graduate Medicine*, 103: 103, 1998.

Kelley, W. N., Harris, E. D., Ruddy, S. *Textbook of Rheumatology*. Philadelphia: W. B. Saunders, 1997.

Lorig, K., Fries, J. F., *The Arthritis Helpbook: A Tested*

Self-Management Program for Coping with Your Arthritis, New York: Addison-Wesley, 1990.

Mottonen, T., Paimela, L., Leirisalo-Repo, M., Kautiainen, H., Ilonen, J., Hannonen, P., "Only high disease activity and positive rheumatoid factor indicate poor prognosis in patients with early rheumatoid arthritis treated with 'sawtooth' strategy," *Annals of Rheumatic Disease*, 57: 533–539, 1998.

Nelson, M. E., "A one-year walking program and increased dietary calcium in post-menopausal women: Effects on bone," *Journal of Clinical Nutrition*, 53: 1304–1311, 1991.

"Notice to Readers: Availability of Lyme Disease Vaccine," *Morbidity and Mortality Weekly Report*, January 22, 1999/48(02); 35–36, 43.

O'Dell, J. R., Pischel, K. D., Weinblatt, M., Glaser, V., "Rheumatoid arthritis: What's new in treatment," *Patient Care*, 31: 5, 1997.

Pisetsky, D. S., Trien, S. F., *The Duke University Medical Center Book of Arthritis*, New York: Fawcett Columbine, 1992.

"Rheumatoid arthritis: Symptoms, diagnosis, and clinical management," *Drug Store News*, September 21, 1998. Shlotzhauer, T. L., McGuire, J. L. *Living with Rheumatoid Arthritis*, Baltimore: The Johns Hopkins University Press, 1993.

Steere, A. C., "Lyme disease," *New England Journal of Medicine*, 321: 586–596, 1989.

van de Putte, L. B. A., van Gestel, A. M., van Riel, P. L. C. M, "Early treatment of rheumatoid arthritis: Rationale, evidence, and implications," *Annals of Rheumatic Disease*, 57: 511–512, 1998.

∾ CHAPTER TWO

Anderson, G. D., Hauser, S. D., McGarity, K. L., Bremer, M. E., Isakson, P. C., Gregory, S. A., "Selective inhibition of cyclooxygenase (COX) 2 reverses inflammation and expression of COX 2 and interleukin 6 in rat adjuvant arthritis," *Journal of Clinical Investigation*, 97: 2672–2679, 1996.

Barner, A., "Review of clinical trials and benefit/risk ratio of meloxicam," *Scandinavian Journal of Rheumatology*, 25 (Suppl 102): 29–37, 1996.

Crofford, L. J., "COX 1 and COX 2 tissue expression: Implications and predictions," *Journal of Rheumatology*, 24 (Suppl 49): 15–19, 1997.

Distal, M., Mueller, C., Bluhmki, E., Fries, J., "Safety of meloxicam: A global analysis of clinical trials," *British Journal of Rheumatology*, 35 (Suppl 1): 68–77.

Emery, P., "Clinical implications of selective cyclooxygenase-2 inhibition," *Scandinavian Journal of Rheumatology*, 25 (Suppl 102): 23–28, 1996.

Furst, D. E., "Meloxicam: Selective COX-2 inhibition in clinical practice," *Seminars in Arthritis and Rheumatology*, 26 (6 Suppl 1): 21–27, 1997.

Furst, D. E., "Perspectives on the cyclooxygenase 2/ cyclooxygenase 1 hypothesis," *Journal of Clinical Rheumatology*, 4 (Suppl): S40–S48, 1998.

Gierse, J. K., McDonald, J. J., Hauser, S. D., Rangwala, S. H., Koboldt, C. M., Seibert, K., "A single amino acid difference between cyclooxygenase 1 (COX 1) and 2 (COX 2) reverses the selectivity of COX-2 specific inhibitors," *Journal of Biological Chemistry*, 271: 15810–15814, 1996.

Huskission, E. C., Ghozlan, R., Kurthen, R., Degner, F. L., Bluhmki, E., "A long-term study to evaluate the safety and efficacy of meloxicam therapy in patients with rheumatoid arthritis," *British Journal of Rheumatology*, 35 (Suppl 1): 29–34, 1996.

Isakson, P. C., "Outcome of specific COX-2 inhibition in rheumatoid arthritis," *Journal of Rheumatology*, 24 (Suppl 49): 9–14, 1997.

Lane, N. E., "Pain management in osteoarthritis: The role of COX-2 inhibitors," *Journal of Rheumatology*, 24 (Suppl 49): 20–24, 1997.

McCann, J., "Arthritis hope; new drugs," *Drug Topics*, 2: 52, 1998.

Needleman, P., presentation at the Workshop on Nitric Oxide and Cyclooxygenase, Florence, Italy, October 15–17, 1998.

Pairet, M., "Pharmacologic characterization of meloxicam," *Journal of Clinical Rheumatology*, 4 (Suppl): S26–S31, 1998.

Reginster, J. Y., Distel, M., Bluhmki, E., "A double-blind, three-week study to compare the efficacy and safety of meloxicam 7.5 mg and meloxicam 15 mg in patients with rheumatoid arthritis," *British Journal of Rheumatology*, 35 (Suppl 1): 17–21, 1996.

Seibert, K., Zhang, Y., Leahy, K., Hauser, S., Masferrer, J., Perkins, W., "Pharmacological and biochemical demonstration of the role of cyclooxygenase 2 in inflammation and pain," *Proceedings of the National Academy of Science, USA*, 91: 12013–12017, 1994.

Simon, L. S., Lanza, F. L., Lipsky, P. E., Hubbard, R. C., Talwalker, S., Schwartz, B. D., Isakson, P. C., Geis, G. S., "Preliminary study of the safety and efficacy of SC-58635, a novel cyclooxygenase-2 inhibitor: Efficacy and safety in two placebo-controlled trials in osteoarthritis and rheumatoid arthritis, and studies of gastrointestinal and platelet effects," *Arthritis and Rheumatology*, 41: 1591–1602, 1998.

Wojtulewski, J. A., Schattenkirchner, M., Barcelo, P., LeLoet, X., Bevis, P. J., Bluhmki, E., Distel, M., "A six-month, double-blind trial to compare the efficacy and safety of meloxicam 7.5 mg daily and naproxen 750 mg daily in patients with rheumatoid arthritis," *British Journal of Rheumatology*, 35 (Suppl 1): 22–28, 1996.

Wolfe, Y. L., "Guard your gut: Upcoming drug seeks gentler arthritis relief," *Prevention*, 2: 53, 1997.

∾ CHAPTER THREE

ACR Clinical Guidelines Committee, "Guidelines for the management of rheumatoid arthritis," *Arthritis and Rheumatism*, 39: 713–722, 1996.

Brooks, P., "Rheumatology," *British Medical Journal*, 316: 1810, 1998.

Dunkin, M. A., "Drug guide," *Arthritis Today*, 1997.

Evans, C., presentation at the Workshop on Nitric Oxide and Cyclooxygenase, Florence, Italy, October 15–17, 1998.

Fries, J., "The epidemiology of NSAID gastropathy: The ARAMIS experience," *Journal of Clinical Rheumatology*, 4 (Suppl): S11–S16, 1998.

Fries, J., "Toward an understanding of NSAID-related adverse events: The contribution of longitudinal data," *Scandinavian Journal of Rheumatology*, 25 (Suppl 102): 3–8, 1996.

Furst, D. E., "Perspectives on the cyclooxygenase 2/ cyclooxygenase 1 hypothesis," *Journal of Clinical Rheumatology*, 4 (Suppl): S40–S48, 1998.

Gierse, J. K., McDonald, J. J., Hauser, S. D., Rangwala, S. H., Koboldt, C. M., Seibert, K., "A single amino acid difference between cyclooxygenase 1 (COX 1) and 2 (COX 2) reverses the selectivity of COX-2 specific inhibitors," *Journal of Biological Chemistry*, 271: 15810–15814, 1996.

Kurumbail, R. G., Stevens, A. M., Gierse, J. K., McDonald, J. J., Stegeman, R. A., Pak, J. Y., Gildehaus, D., Miyashiro, J. M., Penning, T. D., Seibert, K., Isakson, P. C., Stallings, W. C., "Structural basis for selective inhibition of cyclooxygenase 2 by anti-inflammatory agents," *Nature*, 384: 644–648, 1996.

O'Dell, J. R., Pischel, K. D., Weinblatt, M., Glaser, V., "Rheumatoid arthritis: What's new in treatment," *Patient Care*, 31: 5, 1997.

"On the trail of new arthritis treatments," *Harvard Health Letter*, 1: 7, 1997.

Portanova, J. P., Zhang, Y., Anderson, G. D., Hauser, S. D., Masferrer, J. L., Seibert, K., Gregory, S. A., Isakson, P. C., "Selective neutralization of prostaglandin E_2 blocks inflammation, hyperalgesia, and interleukin 6 production in vivo," *Journal of Experimental Medicine*, 184: 883–891, 1996.

Portyansky, E., "Hitting RA head-on," *Drug Topics*, 17: 21, 1998.

"Rheumatoid arthritis: Symptoms, diagnosis, and clinical management," *Drug Store News*, September 21, 1998.

Seibert, K., Zhang, Y., Leahy, K., Hauser, S., Masferrer, J., Perkins, W., Lee, L., Isakson, P., "Pharmacological and biochemical demonstration of the role of cyclooxygenase 2 in inflammation and pain," *Proceedings of the National Academy of Science, USA*, 91: 12013–12017, 1994.

van de Putte, L. B. A., van Gestel, A. M., van Riel, P. L. C. M, "Early treatment of rheumatoid arthritis: Rationale, evidence, and implications," *Annals of Rheumatic Disease*, 57: 511–512, 1998.

Vane, J. R., "Differential inhibition of cyclooxygenase isoforms. An explanation of the action of NSAIDs," *Journal of Clinical Rheumatology*, 4 (Suppl): S3–S10, 1998.

Vane, J. R., Botting, R. M., "Mechanism of action of anti-inflammatory drugs," *Scandinavian Journal of Rheumatology*, 25 (Suppl 102): 9–21, 1996.

∾ CHAPTER FOUR

Barner, A., "Review of clinical trials and benefit/risk ratio of meloxicam," *Scandinavian Journal of Rheumatology*, 25 (Suppl 102): 29–37, 1996.

Distel, M., "Meloxicam: Clinical data on a preferential cyclooxygenase-2 inhibitor," *Journal of Clinical Rheumatology*, 4 (Suppl): S32–S39, 1998.

Distel, M., Mueller, C., Bluhmki, E., Fries, J., "Safety of meloxicam: A global analysis of clinical trials," *British Journal of Rheumatology*, 35 (Suppl 1): 68–77.

Emery, P., "Clinical implications of selective cyclooxygenase-2 inhibition," *Scandinavian Journal of Rheumatology*, 25 (Suppl 102): 23–28, 1996.

Furst, D. E., "Meloxicam: Selective COX-2 inhibition in clinical practice," *Seminars in Arthritis and Rheumatology*, 26 (6 Suppl 1): 21–27, 1997.

Geis, G. S., Hubbard, R., Callison, D., Yu, S., Zhao, W., "Safety and efficacy of celecoxib, a specific COX-2 inhibitor, in patients with rheumatoid arthritis," Presented at the 62nd meeting of the American College of Rheumatology, San Diego, CA, November 8–12, 1998.

Hubbard, R., Geis, G. S., Woods, E., Yu, S., Zhao, W., "Efficacy, tolerability, and safety of celecoxib, a specific COX-2 inhibitor, in osteoarthritis," Presented at the 62nd meeting of the American College of Rheumatology, San Diego, CA, November 8–12, 1998.

Huskission, E. C., Ghozlan, R., Kurthen, R., Degner, F. L., Bluhmki, E., "A long-term study to evaluate the safety and efficacy of meloxicam therapy in patients with rheumatoid arthritis," *British Journal of Rheumatology*, 35 (Suppl 1): 29–34, 1996.

Isakson, P. C., "Outcome of specific COX-2 inhibition in rheumatoid arthritis," *Journal of Rheumatology*, 24 (Suppl 49): 9–14, 1997.

Karim, A., Tolbert, D., Piergies, A., Hunt, T., Hubbard, R., Harper, K., Slater, M., Geis, G. S., "Celecoxib, a specific COX-2 inhibitor, lacks significant drug-drug interactions with methotrexate or warfarin," Presented at the 62nd meeting of the American College of Rheumatology, San Diego, CA, November 8–12, 1998.

Lane, N. E., "Pain management in osteoarthritis: The role of COX-2 inhibitors," *Journal of Rheumatology*, 24 (Suppl 49): 20–24, 1997.

Masferrer, J. L., Zweifel, B. S., Manning, P. T., et al., "Selective inhibition of inducible cyclooxygenase 2 in vivo is anti-inflammatory and nonulcerogenic,'' *Proceedings of the National Academy of Science, USA*, 91: 3228–3232, 1994.

McCann, J., ''Arthritis hope; new drugs,'' *Drug Topics*, 2: 52, 1998.

Pairet, M., ''Inhibition of cyclooxygenase 1 and cyclooxygenase 2: Analysis of in vitro test systems and their clinical relevance,'' *Journal of Clinical Rheumatology*, 4 (Suppl): S17–S25, 1998.

Pairet, M., ''Pharmacologic characterization of meloxicam,'' *Journal of Clinical Rheumatology*, 4 (Suppl): S26–S31, 1998.

Reginster, J. Y., Distel, M., Bluhmki, E., ''A double-blind, three-week study to compare the efficacy and safety of meloxicam 7.5 mg and meloxicam 15 mg in patients with rheumatoid arthritis,'' *British Journal of Rheumatology*, 35 (Suppl 1): 17–21, 1996.

Simon, L. S., Lanza, F. L., Lipsky, P. E., Hubbard, R. C., Talwalker, S., Schwartz, B. D., Isakson, P. C., Geis, G. S., ''Preliminary study of the safety and efficacy of SC-58635, a novel cyclooxygenase-2 inhibitor: Efficacy and safety in two placebo-controlled trials in osteoarthritis and rheumatoid arthritis, and studies of gastrointestinal and platelet effects,'' *Arthritis and Rheumatology*, 41: 1591–1602, 1998.

Weissman, G., presentation at the Workshop on Nitric Oxide and Cyclooxygenase, Florence, Italy, October 15–17, 1998.

Wojtulewski, J. A., Schattenkirchner, M., Barcelo, P., LeLoet, X., Bevis, P. J., Bluhmki, E., Distel, M., ''A six-month, double-blind, trial to compare the efficacy and safety of meloxicam 7.5 mg daily and naproxen

750 mg daily in patients with rheumatoid arthritis,'' *British Journal of Rheumatology*, 35 (Suppl 1): 22–28, 1996.

Wolfe, Y.L., ''Guard your gut: Upcoming drug seeks gentler arthritis relief,'' *Prevention*, 2: 53, 1997.

∾ CHAPTER FIVE

The Arthritis Foundation, *Rheumatoid Arthritis*, Arthritis Foundation brochure.

Pennisi, E. ''Building a better aspirin,'' *Science*, May 22, 1998.

∾ CHAPTER SIX

Arthritis Today, September/October, 1998.

Crofford, L. J., ''COX 1 and COX 2 tissue expression: Implications and predictions,'' *Journal of Rheumatology*, 24 (Suppl 49): 15–19, 1997.

Distel, M., ''Meloxicam: Clinical data on a preferential cyclooxygenase-2 inhibitor,'' *Journal of Clinical Rheumatology*, 4 (Suppl): S32–S39, 1998.

Eberhart, C. E., Coffey, R. J., Radhika, A., Giardiello, F. M., Ferrenbach, S., DuBois, R. N., ''Up-regulation of cyclooxygenase 2 gene expression in human colorectal adenomas and adenocarcinomas,'' *Gastroenterology*, 107: 1183–1188, 1994.

Kargman, S. L., O'Neill, G. P., Vickers, P. J., Evans, J. F., Mancini, J. A., Jothy, S., ''Expression of prostaglandin G/H synthase 1 and 2 protein in human colon cancer,'' *Cancer Research*, 55: 2556–2559, 1995.

Pairet, M., "Pharmacologic characterization of meloxicam," *Journal of Clinical Rheumatology*, 4 (Suppl): S26–S31, 1998.

Pennisi, E., "Building a better aspirin," *Science*, May 22, 1998.

Reddy, B. S., Rao, C. V., Seibert, K., "Evaluation of cyclooxygenase-2 inhibitor for potential chemopreventative properties in colon carcinogenesis," *Cancer Research*, 56: 4566–4569, 1996.

Sheng, H., Shao, J., Kirkland, S. C., et al., "Inhibition of human colon cancer cell growth by selective inhibition of cyclooxygenase 2," *Journal of Clinical Investigation*, 99: 2254–2259, 1997.

Stewart, W. F., Kawas, C., Corrada, M., Metter, E. J., "Risk of Alzheimer's disease and duration of NSAID use," *Neurology*, 48: 626–632, 1997.

Vane, J. R., "Differential inhibition of cyclooxygenase isoforms: An explanation of the action of NSAIDs," *Journal of Clinical Rheumatology*, 4 (Suppl): S3–S10, 1998.

Yamagata, K., Andreasson, K. I., Kaufmann, W. E., Barnes, C. A., Worley, P. F., "Expression of a mitogen-inducible cyclooxygenase in brain neurons: Regulation of synaptic activity and glucocorticoids," *Neuron*, 11: 371–386, 1993.

∽ CHAPTER SEVEN

"FDA approves new anti-TNF," *Applied Genetics News*, October, 1998.

Furst, D. E., "Perspectives on the cyclooxygenase 2/

cyclooxygenase 1 hypothesis," *Journal of Clinical Rheumatology*, 4 (Suppl): S40–S48, 1998.

O'Dell, J. R., Pischel, K. D., Weinblatt, M., Glaser, V., "Rheumatoid arthritis: What's new in treatment," *Patient Care*, 31: 5, 1997.

Sadovsky, R., "New treatment strategies for rheumatoid arthritis," *American Family Physician*, 4: 1185, 1997.

Ziegler, J., "New NSAID for arthritis is kinder, gentler on stomach," *Drug Topics*, 23: 32, 1997.

◌ CHAPTER EIGHT

The Arthritis Foundation, *Arthritis Answers*, Arthritis Foundation brochure.

The Arthritis Foundation, *Arthritis 101*, Marietta, GA: Longstreet Press, 1997.

The Arthritis Foundation, *Exercise and Your Arthritis*, Arthritis Foundation brochure.

The Arthritis Foundation, *Managing Your Activities*, Arthritis Foundation brochure.

Lorig, K., Fries, J. F., *The Arthritis Helpbook: A Tested Self-Management Program for Coping with Your Arthritis*. New York: Addison-Wesley, 1990.

Pisetsky, D. S., Trien, S. F. *The Duke University Medical Center Book of Arthritis*, New York: Fawcett Columbine, 1992.

Ross, I., "Does Your HMO Work for You?", *Reader's Digest*, 29–36, November, 1998.

Shlotzhauer, T. L., McGuire, J. L. *Living with Rheumatoid Arthritis*, Baltimore: The Johns Hopkins University Press, 1993.

Index

A

Acetaminophen, 12, 41, 68, 158
Acetylcholine, 114
Activities of daily living. *See* Daily activities, performing
Acupuncture, 87, 157
Adrenal glands, 65
Aerobic exercise, 147–148
Age, as arthritis factor, 27
AIDS arthritis, 11
Air travel, 168–169
Alcohol consumption, 88, 98, 158
Alendronate, 67
Alternative treatments, 134
  acupuncture and massage, 87, 157
  dietary, 88, 134, 153–154
  herbal remedies, 87–88, 155–156

natural drugs, 87–88
  See also Exercise
Alzheimer's disease
  care and supervision of patients, 113
  Cox-2 inhibitors as protection against, 112, 113, 115
  drug treatment of, 113–115
  symptoms of, 112–113
American Academy of Physical Medicine and Rehabilitation (AAPMR), 197, 203
American College of Rheumatology, 35, 197–198, 207
American Juvenile Arthritis Organization, 201
American Occupational Therapy Association, 207–208

E

F

G

Dr. Robert G. Lahita received his M.D. and Ph.D. from Jefferson Medical College in Philadelphia and did his internship and residency in internal medicine at the New York Hospital in New York City. He completed his fellowship in rheumatology and immunology at Rockefeller Hospital. For many years he served as senior attending physician at St. Luke's-Roosevelt Hospital Center, New York, as well as serving as full-time academic faculty and medical administrator. During this time he was also an Associate Professor at Columbia University College of Physicians and Surgeons in New York City.

Dr. Lahita is now affiliated with New York Medical College and St. Vincent's Medical Center. He is the author of several books on arthritis and related diseases for the lay public as well as for professionals. Dr. Lahita is board certified in Internal Medicine and is a member of the American College of Rheumatology.

Complete and Authoritative
Health Care Books From Wholecare